HOW DRUGS WORK

DRUG ABUSE AND THE HUMAN BODY

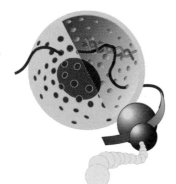

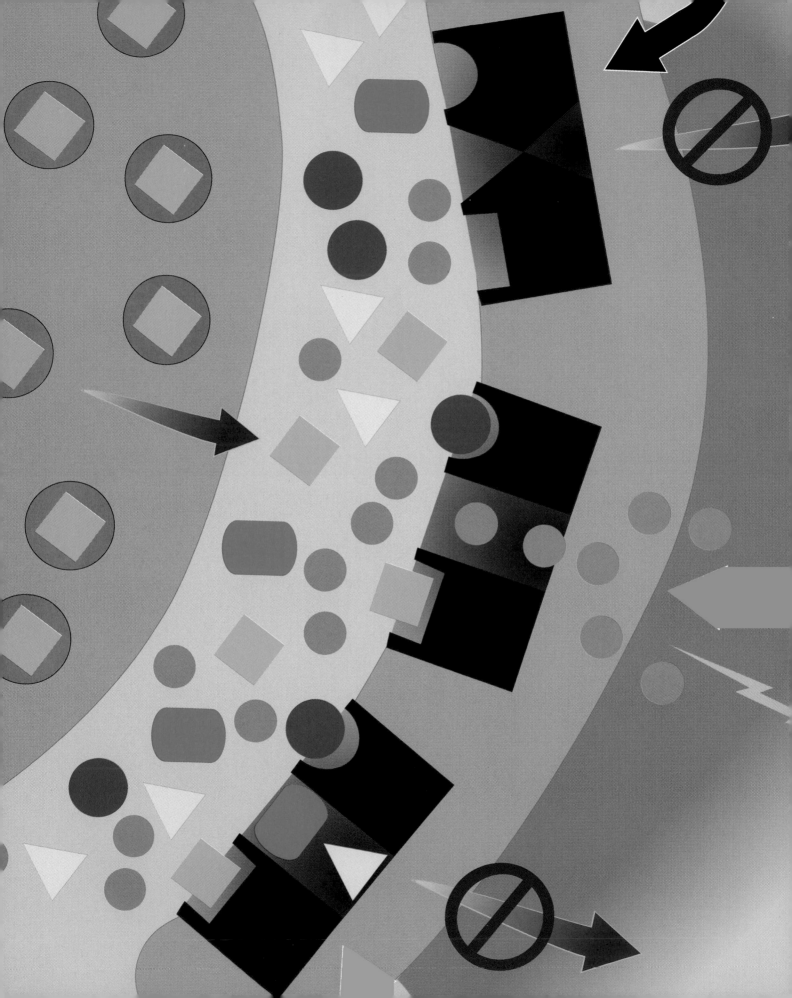

HOW DRUGS WORK

DRUG ABUSE AND THE HUMAN BODY

GESINA L. LONGENECKER, PH.D.

Illustrated by
NELSON W. HEE

Ziff-Davis Press
Emeryville, California

Development Editor	Valerie Haynes Perry
Copy Editor	Kelly Green
Technical Reviewer	Donna K. Curtis, Pharm.D.
Project Coordinator	Barbara Dahl
Proofreader	Carol Burbo
Cover Illustration	Nelson W. Hee and Regan Honda
Cover Design	Carrie English
Book Design	Carrie English
Technical Illustration	Nelson W. Hee
Word Processing	Howard Blechman
Page Layout	Bruce Lundquist
Indexer	Ted Laux

Ziff-Davis Press books are produced on a Macintosh computer system with the following applications: FrameMaker®, Microsoft® Word, QuarkXPress®, Adobe Illustrator®, Adobe Photoshop®, Adobe Streamline™, MacLink®*Plus*, Aldus® FreeHand™, Collage Plus™.

If you have comments or questions or would like to receive a free catalog, call or write:
Ziff-Davis Press
5903 Christie Avenue
Emeryville, CA 94608
1-800-688-0448

ISBN 1-56276-241-9

Manufactured in the United States of America

 This book is printed on paper that contains 50% total recycled fiber of which 20% is de-inked postconsumer fiber.

10 9 8 7 6 5 4 3 2 1

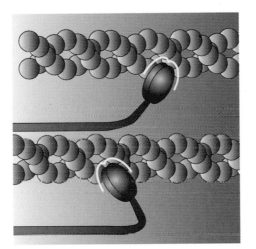

For my parents, who gave
so much for so long, and for
Bart, Gene, Aimee, and Lani,
who put up with me and
encouraged me through
the hard parts.

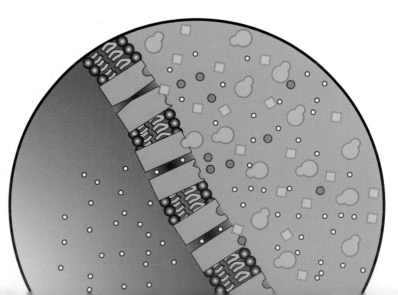

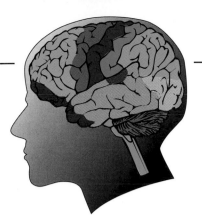
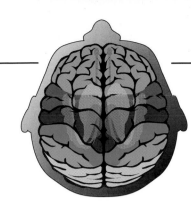

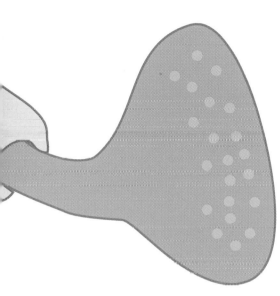

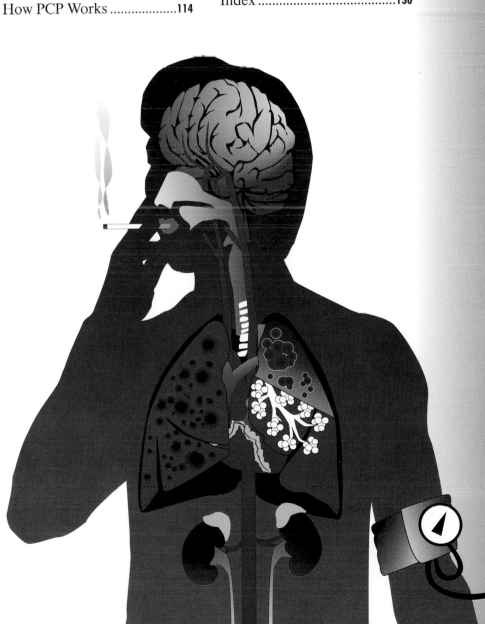

PART 4

Drugs That Alter Mood, Perception, and Image
92

I am grateful to the management of Ziff-Davis Press, especially Cindy Hudson and Eric Stone, for their willingness to allow me to address a longtime goal; they believed this project was possible in my hands and, in their believing, made it real. Throughout, I had expert and patient help from Valerie Perry, development editor: Valerie clarified my prose and streamlined the content to make it do what it was supposed to do. Valerie also coordinated and integrated Donna Curtis's technical reviews and Nelson Hee's graphics. Nelson translated rudimentary sketches and comments into the colorful and communicative graphics that accompany each chapter. Many others at Ziff-Davis, including Kelly Green, Barbara Dahl, Bruce Lundquist, Howard Blechman, and Cori Pansarasa, also contributed to the successful completion of this project.

There were times when an extra little bit of information was needed. Willing and gracious (and occasionally heroic) help was provided by the librarians at the University of South Alabama, by Greg Mitchell of the DEA Office of the Chief Counsel, by Joy Turner of the Mobile Drug Education Council, and by numerous others. Their help made writing this book much easier!

Opportunities to say thanks are rare. A long time ago, a young faculty member at Tulane Medical School was willing to allow a high-school student to work in his lab for a summer. That summer's introduction to pharmacology became a lifelong interest, thanks to Paul Guth. The training to go with the interest resulted from the faith of Walter Riker and an investment by Amir Askari. To both, thanks! This project is yours as much as mine.

Most people are aware of the numerous health, economic, and other problems that are associated with drug abuse. However, many are less aware of the actual effects of abused drugs and know even less about how the effects occur: *How Drugs Work* focuses specifically on these two issues.

The ways in which drugs produce effects on the body follow general principles. The first section of this book introduces you to these principles. After drugs enter the body, they must successfully overcome some bodily defenses in order to ultimately arrive at the location where they take effect. The brain is the main site of action for drugs that are abused. When undesirable effects occur at sites other than the brain, these effects are commonly called side effects.

Different drugs of abuse may interact with different areas of the brain. However, most of these drugs produce effects in one very important brain system: the reward circuit. Pleasure is the reward that drug effects provide in this area of the brain. Once this pleasure is experienced, it serves as some of the motivation for continued drug use. The reward circuit is an important part of our survival. It is ordinarily activated by such common behaviors as eating.

Once you understand the mechanisms of drug abuse, it will be easier for you to follow discussions about the various categories of drugs. You will learn about differences and similarities between drugs that alter mood, perception, and image. You will also discover some interesting facts about drugs that are classified as stimulants or depressants. For example, did you know that a narcotic is a specific type of depressant? The term narcotic is frequently used to describe drugs in general even though it belongs to this particular category.

Drug effects in the brain, and elsewhere, most often occur when drugs interact with special cellular structures called receptors. Receptors are part of the body's internal communications system. Different parts of the body communicate via chemical messages, whether the communications are between cells that are close to one another or very far apart. The chemical messages sent by one cell are received by another when the chemical combines with its specific receptors. Cells respond to various messages in one of two ways. The cell is either stimulated, which *increases* its function, or the cell is inhibited, which *decreases* its function.

Many of the chemical messages that the brain receives are known as neurotransmitters. Some drugs have a chemical structure similar to the body's naturally occurring chemical messages, including the neurotransmitters. This book explains how these drugs cause effects by interacting with the receptors for the neurotransmitter they resemble. Narcotics, amphetamine, and LSD are examples of drugs that fall into this category.

Neurotransmitters usually stimulate or inhibit cells. Because drugs can mimic these activities, they can also prevent, or *block*, the effects of neurotransmitters by interacting with certain receptors to prevent a cell from accessing a message. Furthermore, if a drug *blocks* the effect of an *inhibitory* message, then the effect of the drug may appear to be stimulation. The opposite is also true: a drug that blocks a stimulatory message appears to be an inhibitor. You will become familiar with these interactions as you read this book.

Chemical messages such as neurotransmitters and drugs can interact in several other ways as well. For example, stimulation and inhibition of cells are both stopped when the message is removed. This usually occurs either when an enzyme breaks down the message or when the message is returned to the cell from which it was sent. The latter process, called re-uptake, is fairly common for neurotransmitters. The illustrations in this book clearly depict this process. Drugs can decrease breakdown or limit re-uptake and thus change the duration and intensity of neurotransmitter effect. Cocaine is an excellent example of a drug that inhibits re-uptake of several neurotransmitters. The effects of cocaine are really the effects of increased amounts of neurotransmitter acting on cells for a longer period of time than usual.

The many effects that drugs of abuse have on the body will become increasingly apparent as you read this book. The similarities in how these effects occur will also become clear. What may be most striking is that while drugs of abuse start their effects in different areas of the reward circuit and in different ways, most of them ultimately stimulate it. An awareness of the general patterns of these effects will help the reader understand the effects of other drugs as well.

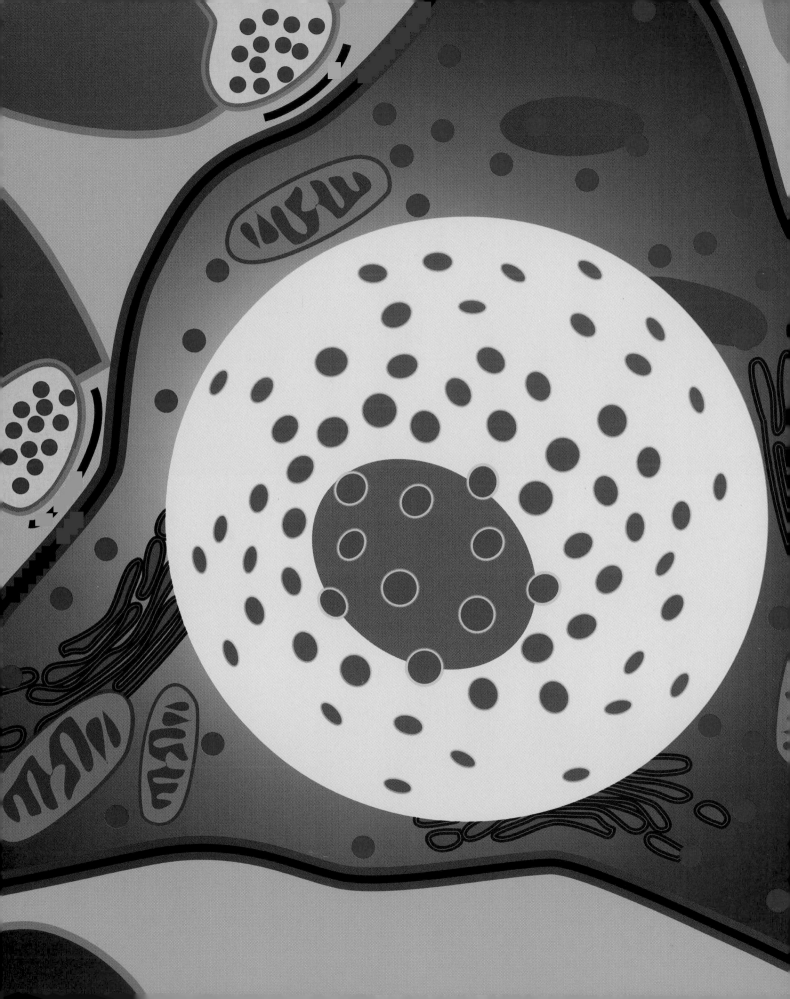

THE MECHANISMS OF DRUG ABUSE

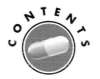

CONTENTS

THIS BOOK IS specifically about drugs that are abused. Almost everyone is familiar with drugs in one of two contexts: drugs a physician prescribes to be taken for health-related reasons, or drugs that are self-administered and abused for reasons unrelated to health. The former context is a societally-accepted, and thus legal, use, while the latter use is evident but often unsanctioned or even illegal.

A drug is most simply defined as a chemical that causes an effect on a living system. There are pharmacological and toxicological implications of this expanded definition. Pharmacology and toxicology are two related branches of medical science that deal with the study of the effects of chemicals on living systems. Pharmacology is concerned with chemicals that cause desirable effects. Toxicology is more broadly concerned with effects of all chemicals, whether useful or harmful.

The basic definition of a drug is often modified to also state that drugs, in contrast to other chemicals, cause *desirable* or useful effects. Desirability is a very subjective, individual value that does not allow discrimination of medical and nonmedical uses. What, then, distinguishes use from abuse?

There are several important characteristics of legal drugs and sanctioned drug use. First, the drug is usually used to improve health in some way, such as adjusting blood pressure to a value within a range considered normal. Second, the drug has been reviewed and approved for the use through a lengthy process prescribed and overseen by government agencies. The review and approval process assures that the drug acts in the manner claimed by its developer and that it does so safely. This process also ensures that data about the drug are openly and readily available. These data may include any additional effects associated with the drug, its recommended doses, how it should be administered and how often, whether it interacts with other drugs, and so on. The actual preparations of the drug are also standardized, so that the prescriber and consumer know exactly what and how much is being taken.

On the other hand, drug abuse is summarily defined as the self-administration of drugs for reasons unrelated to improving one's health. Drug abuse also carries a connotation of detriment to society, even where legality is not an issue. For example, use of tobacco is not illegal due to an acceptance process that has been described as domestication. This means the use of tobacco became accepted as a matter of individual choice before its real consequences were fully recognized. Its abuse is so widespread at this point that overt legal restriction would be difficult at best. As a result, society has adopted a sort of out-of-sight, out-of-mind approach as a means of encouraging limits on use. More emphasis is being placed on education as a means of making the public conscious of health consequences. Decreased awareness is another method of reducing the acceptance and appeal of using tobacco. Limitation of advertising seeks to achieve this goal.

The review process summarized above for legal, medically useful drugs requires development of methods to detect and determine levels of the drug in various body fluids and tissues. If a drug has not been through such a process, there may be no method for detecting its presence in the body. Therefore, it may be difficult to interpret symptoms for some drugs of abuse, even those from overdoses. In fact, treatment of symptoms resulting from consuming unfamiliar abused drugs may be unavailable or simply not provided.

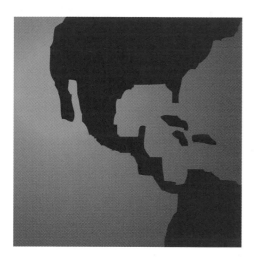

CHAPTER 1

The Origins of Drug Use

ALTHOUGH IT CANNOT be proved, we can surmise that human beings' interest in drugs is as old as self-interest itself, which has endured since our species first came into existence. Indeed, self-consciousness may be our most unique feature. A direct result of this inward focus is an ongoing quest to modify thoughts and sensations, particularly those that are in any way unpleasant.

Early experience with drugs was gained accidentally through consumption of drug-containing plants. Ingesting these plants clearly and emphatically demonstrated that it was possible to relieve pain, dispel fear or perhaps even see the face of God through this quick and easy practice. Favorable initial drug experiences motivated early consumers to identify and remember the drug's source. At first this probably meant that an individual could return to an area, find a specific plant, and repeat the desired experience.

The ability of humans to learn and to provide for themselves led to knowledge and use of an increasingly larger number of drugs. Early consumers also became adept at methods of collecting, preserving, cultivating, and recording the sources of drugs as well as noting their various effects. Different methods of consuming the drugs were developed such as infusions or teas, and the results of such experiments were duly recorded. Drugs were assigned names that often indicated the magic they were intended to induce. For example, the word *chandra* means moon in Hindi. The drug, chandra, was used to treat lunacy, a disorder believed to be caused by the moon. Drugs were less commonly identified by type, classification, or source, at least until later times.

The process of discovering and dispensing started by ordinary individuals evolved into a specialty. Drug specialists achieved positions of power and influence by using and guarding their knowledge: They became the healers, priests, and politicians. These specialists became associated with healing, relief from fear or depression, and blessings from various deities, sometimes through drug-induced euphoria and visions. These powers guaranteed them a high social position. These specialists also provided invaluable legacies in the form of written records, which are still useful today.

Descriptions and lists of drugs, and instructions for their appropriate preparation and administration, are among the oldest written documents. These documents provide the foundation of modern pharmacology as well as offer insights into human history. Suprisingly, many of the drugs in these ancient documents are neither unfamiliar nor outdated. For example, digitalis is one drug preparation that may appear in both the Chinese Pen Tsao and the Egyptian Ebers Papyrus. The indications for use of digitalis in these documents are consistent with symptoms of congestive heart failure: Digitalis drugs are still the mainstay of therapy for congestive heart failure.

However, the digitalis drugs in use today are no longer the native compounds found in nature. Modern pharmacologists study in detail the chemical structure of native compounds. They also identify and study the structures (receptors) on cells with which the drugs interact. Pharmacologists then determine what changes in cell functions occur as a result of using the drug. Using this information, new drugs, related chemically to the natural drug, may be created. These new drugs may be adjusted in ways that provide greater or more specific activity.

Many of the drugs to be discussed in subsequent chapters are extracted directly from nature and have been in use for a long time. However, in most cases the active principle has been isolated and identified for common use. Other drugs that will be covered are purely synthetic. Some synthetic drugs are listed at the bottom left of the figure showing world origins of natural drugs.

Human nature is often blamed for negative behavior. When we consider some of the characteristics of human behavior, drug abuse is a predictable accompaniment to drug use. Curiosity, pleasure, control, and the desire for relief are just a few of these characteristics. The effectiveness of some drugs can easily lead to the "more is better" assumption, which will in turn result in drug abuse. Many of the drugs of abuse that will be discussed in this book have been known for hundreds and even thousands of years. However, abuse as the extensive problem with which we are concerned today is relatively recent: In fact, a critical dividing line occurs around A.D. 1500. The reasons cited for lack of widespread abuse prior to this time include limited availability, weak preparations, and high costs. For example, even though Noah's drunkenness is noted in the Bible, alcohol abuse was limited in ancient times. This was due to the relatively low amounts of alcohol that can be created in naturally fermented beers and wines (less than 10% and less than 20%, respectively). Distillation was introduced about A.D. 1250, allowing for creation of beverages with alcohol contents that often exceeded 50%. However, despite availability, costs of such beverages were out of reach of most until after 1500; the first instances of widespread abuse were reported in England during the period 1525 to 1550.

Smoking was introduced throughout the world subsequent to the discovery of the Americas. Smoking allows high amounts of a drug to be absorbed via high-concentration delivery to the extremely large surface area of the lungs, which also have a very high blood flow. Opium was smoked until the hypodermic syringe was introduced in 1853. This new method of administering opium significantly affected the impact of the active principles of opium and Coca, which are morphine and cocaine. The use of hypodermic syringes launched direct intravenous administration of drugs.

Recently introduced drugs have little to impede their entry into the abuse scene, as evidenced by the case of phencyclidine (PCP). PCP was introduced in the late 1950s and was already heavily abused by 1970, barely over 10 years later.

World Contributions to Drugs of Abuse

Shown here are the drug, its most common botanical source, the active ingredient(s), and the approximate date of introduction or documented use.

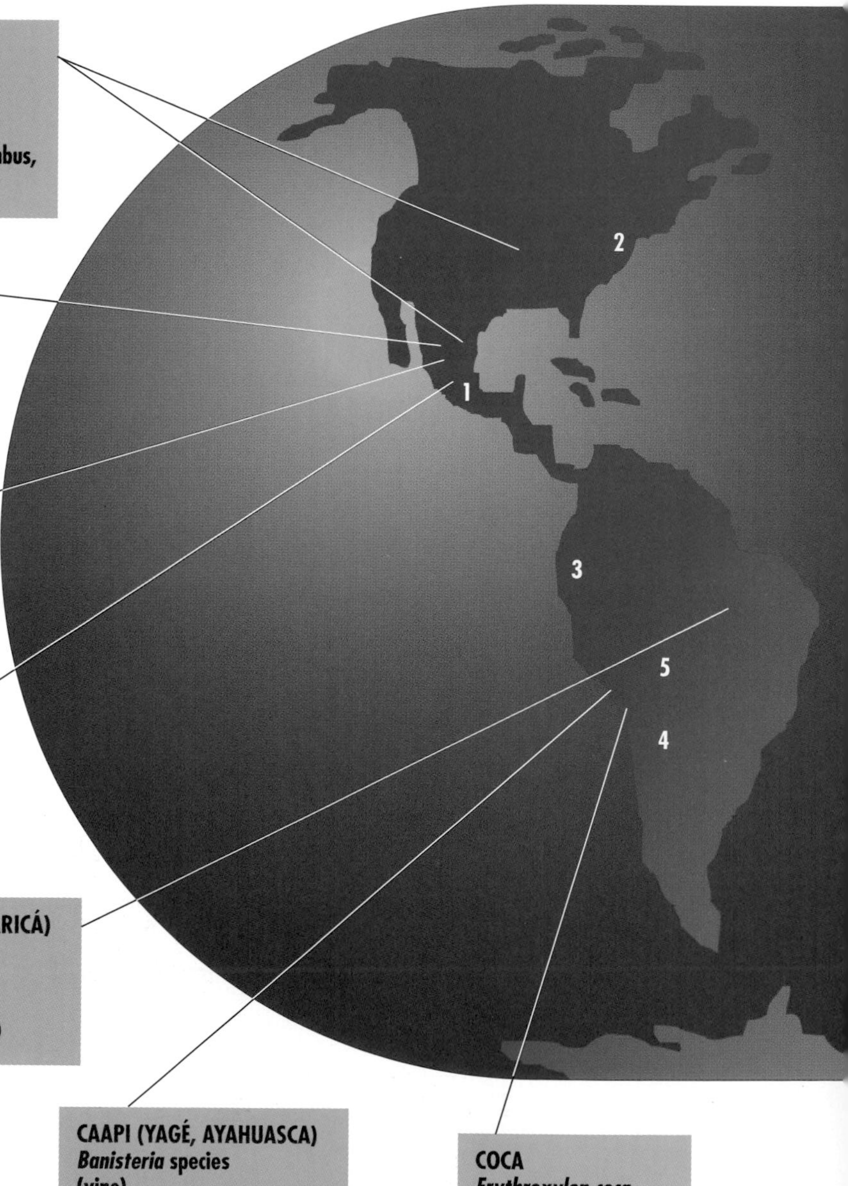

TOBACCO
Nicotiana tabacum, rusticana
(herbaceous plant)
nicotine
earlier than 1492, at discovery by Columbus, other Spanish explorers

PEYOTE
Lophophora williamsii
(cactus)
mescaline
earlier than 300 B.C.

CAFFEINE
(all earlier than A.D.1500):
1. COCOA (*Theobroma cacao*)
2. CASSINA (*Ilex vomitoria*)
   earlier than A.D. 1492
3. WAYUS (*Ilex quayesa*)
4. MATE (*Ilex paraguayensis*)
5. GUARANA (*Paullinea sorbilis*)
6. TEA (*Thea sinensis*)
   circa 2700 B.C.
7. COFFEE (*Coffea arabica*)
   circa A.D. 500
8. KOLA (*Cola nitida*)

OLOLIUQUI
Rivea corymbosa
(morning glory vine)
lysergic acid amide
earlier than A.D. 1500

TEONANACATL
Psilocybe mexicana
(mushroom)
psilocybin, psilocin
earlier than A.D. 1500

SYNTHETICS (not shown):
ETHER (1543)
AMPHETAMINE (1887)
METHAMPETAMINE (1919)
BARBITAL (1903)
SYSERGIC ACID DIETHYLAMIDE (1938)
PHENCYCLIDINE (1955)
TESTOSTERONE (1935)

COHOBA (NIOPO, PARICÁ)
Piptadenia peregrina
(tree)
bufotenin
earlier than A.D. 1500

CAAPI (YAGÉ, AYAHUASCA)
Banisteria species
(vine)
harmine
earlier than A.D. 1500

COCA
Erythroxylon coca
(shrub, tree)
cocaine
earlier than 1500 B.C.

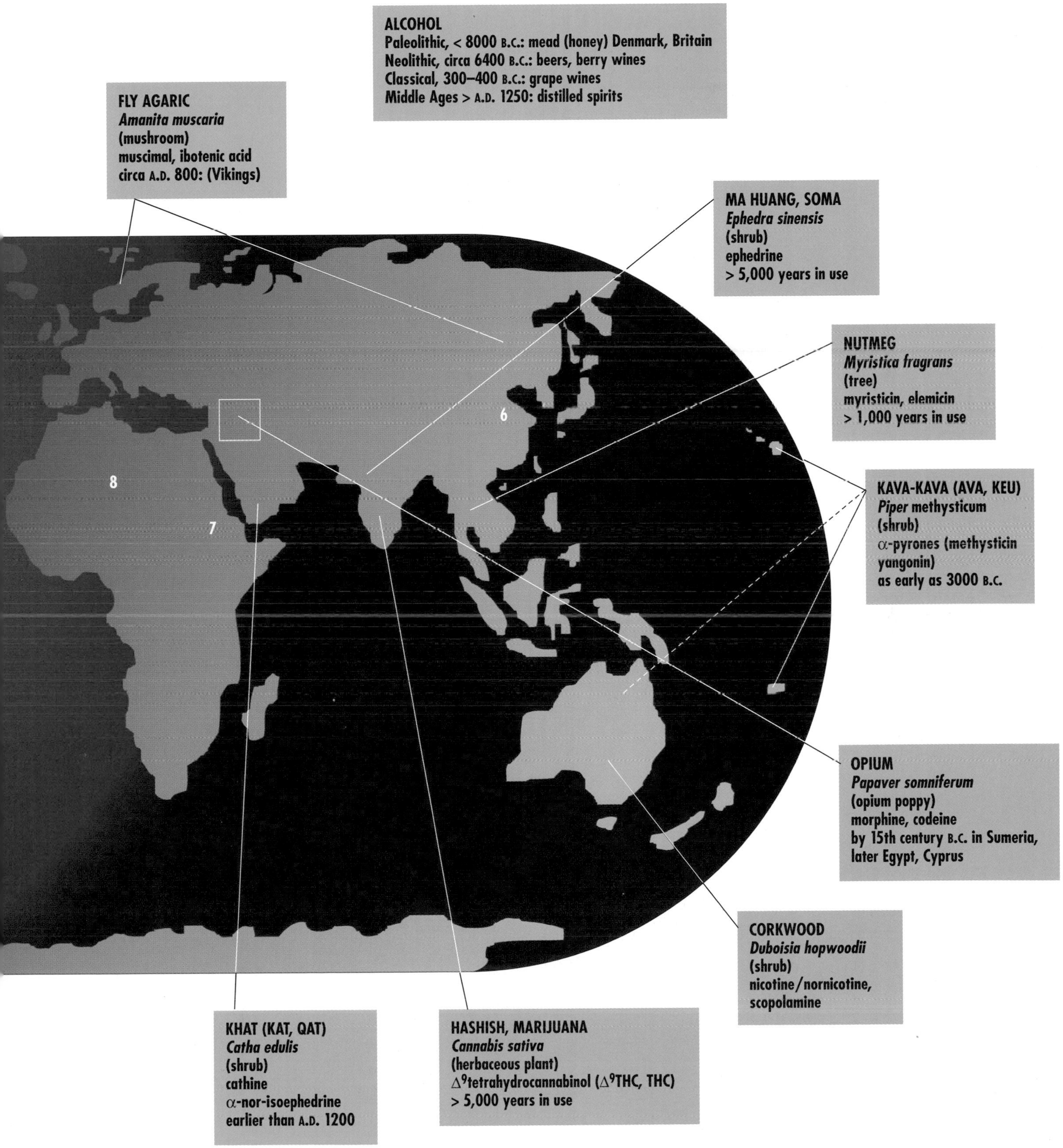

ALCOHOL
Paleolithic, < 8000 B.C.: mead (honey) Denmark, Britain
Neolithic, circa 6400 B.C.: beers, berry wines
Classical, 300–400 B.C.: grape wines
Middle Ages > A.D. 1250: distilled spirits

FLY AGARIC
Amanita muscaria
(mushroom)
muscimal, ibotenic acid
circa A.D. 800: (Vikings)

MA HUANG, SOMA
Ephedra sinensis
(shrub)
ephedrine
> 5,000 years in use

NUTMEG
Myristica fragrans
(tree)
myristicin, elemicin
> 1,000 years in use

KAVA-KAVA (AVA, KEU)
Piper methysticum
(shrub)
α-pyrones (methysticin
yangonin)
as early as 3000 B.C.

OPIUM
Papaver somniferum
(opium poppy)
morphine, codeine
by 15th century B.C. in Sumeria,
later Egypt, Cyprus

CORKWOOD
Duboisia hopwoodii
(shrub)
nicotine/nornicotine,
scopolamine

KHAT (KAT, QAT)
Catha edulis
(shrub)
cathine
α-nor-isoephedrine
earlier than A.D. 1200

HASHISH, MARIJUANA
Cannabis sativa
(herbaceous plant)
△⁹tetrahydrocannabinol (△⁹THC, THC)
> 5,000 years in use

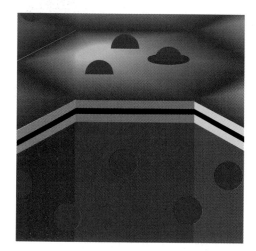

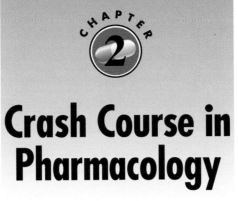

Crash Course in Pharmacology

PHARMACOLOGY IS A science that considers the effects of specific drugs or chemicals on biological systems. It is one of the younger medical sciences, and it was founded by the German scientist Paul Ehrlich just over a hundred years ago. The development of pharmacology resulted from Ehrlich's search for a "magic bullet" that would cure syphilis without simultaneously killing the patient. This pharmacological objective is known as selective toxicity. As the single most important principle of pharmacology, *selective toxicity* contends that the ideal drug should yield only the desired effect and no others. Very few drugs approach this ideal.

Drugs fall into two large categories: There are agonists and antagonists. *Agonists* produce effects, and *antagonists* block the effects of hormones and other chemicals in the body, as well as other drugs. Drugs are further grouped by the type of effect that is produced or blocked, such as depressants or antidepressants. Type-of-effect groups can be further divided according to how the effect is produced. In general, a drug produces effects because it resembles a body chemical and interacts with the structures, or receptors, on cells that are intended for the actual body chemical. The drug-receptor interaction either triggers or prevents a sequence of biochemical changes that ultimately changes the function of the cell, tissue, and/or organ.

Drugs can be taken in many ways. They can be taken orally, by inhalation into the lungs, by inhalation into the nose, and by injection. Some routes are easier and safer than others. The route of administration can influence the likelihood that a drug with abuse potential will actually be abused. For example, smoking opium was introduced throughout the world in the sixteenth century. This route of administration helped raise opium (morphine) use in China to a problem status. Injection, including intravenous injection, became possible with the invention of the hypodermic syringe during the time of the U.S. Civil War. Intravenous injection resulted in significant morphine and cocaine dependence and abuse in the latter part of the last century, before the abuse potential related to this route was really understood. These two routes, smoking and intravenous injection, have had a major impact on drug abuse.

Drugs move predictably around the body regardless of the route of administration; the only variables are how long a drug takes to have an effect and how long the effect lasts. A drug administered orally may take longer to produce an effect than the same drug taken intravenously.

However, the effect from the oral route may last significantly longer than that from the intravenous route.

Some drugs can produce undesirable side effects. Side effects can be significant because in some cases they may cause great discomfort, or they may even be life-threatening. For example, morphine can produce euphoria, a pleasant sensory state. However, it can also depress and even stop respiration. Failure to breathe is the fatal side effect of a morphine overdose. Drugs can even cause severe allergic reactions as side effects. Penicillin allergy is a familiar example.

A single drug can be identified in several ways: by its generic name, chemical name, or company name. For example, aspirin is the generic name for the drug whose chemical name is acetylsalicylic acid. And various companies manufacture aspirin. Drugs of abuse usually also have "street" names in addition to their common names. For example, marijuana is also known as *grass* or *pot*.

Information about drugs is available from numerous sources. Drug information in written or electronic form is generally easiest to find using a generic name. Pharmacology textbooks (such as Goodman and Gilman's *Pharmacological Basis of Therapeutics*), compendia (such as *The National Formulary* and *The U. S. Pharmacopeia*), and books on particular drug topics are available in libraries. This is especially true of libraries that are associated with health education and service facilities. The *Physicians Desk Reference* (*PDR*) and several related style manuals are readily available and provide basic information about effects, doses, dose forms, and side effects. Local and state drug education councils, and particularly the National Clearinghouse for Alcohol and Drug Information (1–800–729–6686) are also excellent sources of this type of information.

How Drugs Produce Effects

Drugs mimic normal body chemicals such as hormones. Hormones and drugs signal cells to changes in their environment and cause cell functions to change accordingly.

1 Drugs interact with cells through specialized structures already present for regular functions. In this case, the specialized structure is a surface receptor. Receptors are connected to other cell structures that are important to cell functions. Cells differ in the type and number of receptors they have according to tissue type and environment. Thus, whether a drug can cause an effect on a particular cell and/or tissue is determined by the presence or absence of suitable receptors. The intensity of effect is influenced by the density of the receptors as well as the amount of the drug available.

2 Drugs act as "first messengers" of signals from receptors. The interaction between a drug and a receptor is detected and transmitted to intracellular structures and processes. The receptor and processes are coupled, frequently through G-proteins. G-proteins adjust basic cell functions, amplifying them or modulating them, or even turning them on or off.

3 Receipt and transmission of a signal from a specific receptor coupled to a G-protein might, for example, cause calcium content to increase. Other receptors can use their respective G-proteins to elicit changes in the production of the compound cAMP (cyclic adenosine monophosphate). Calcium (Ca) and cAMP function as "second messengers" and continue the signal transmission process.

4 Adenosine triphosphate (ATP) is an energy storage compound. Hydrolysis of one of its phosphates yields energy that can be used to accomplish other cell functions. *Hydrolysis* involves splitting a molecular bond and adding the elements of water—hydrogen,and oxygen.

Neurotransmitters

Drugs

Surface receptor

Ca

ATP

ATP

Ca

Ca

Ca

"Second messenger"

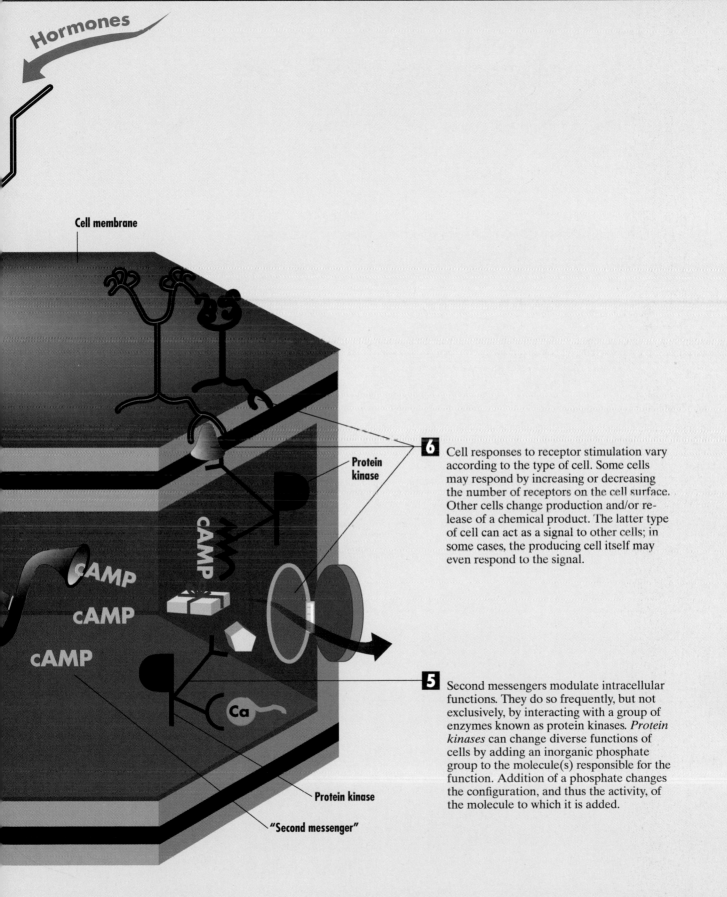

Hormones

Cell membrane

Protein kinase

cAMP

cAMP

cAMP

cAMP

cAMP

Ca

Protein kinase

"Second messenger"

6 Cell responses to receptor stimulation vary according to the type of cell. Some cells may respond by increasing or decreasing the number of receptors on the cell surface. Other cells change production and/or release of a chemical product. The latter type of cell can act as a signal to other cells; in some cases, the producing cell itself may even respond to the signal.

5 Second messengers modulate intracellular functions. They do so frequently, but not exclusively, by interacting with a group of enzymes known as protein kinases. *Protein kinases* can change diverse functions of cells by adding an inorganic phosphate group to the molecule(s) responsible for the function. Addition of a phosphate changes the configuration, and thus the activity, of the molecule to which it is added.

How Drugs Get from Here to There

The individual cell is the basic unit of the body. Each cell is surrounded by a membrane. Drugs must cross the cell membrane many times to be absorbed and distributed to a site of effect. This process must also continue in order to pass along the drug to sites of elimination and excretion after a dose is administered.

A drug moves from high-to low-concentration sites. Most drugs cross membranes by dissolving in the lipids (fats) of the membranes. Occasionally, special carrier molecules help drugs cross membranes. These molecules are typically used by naturally occurring body chemicals.

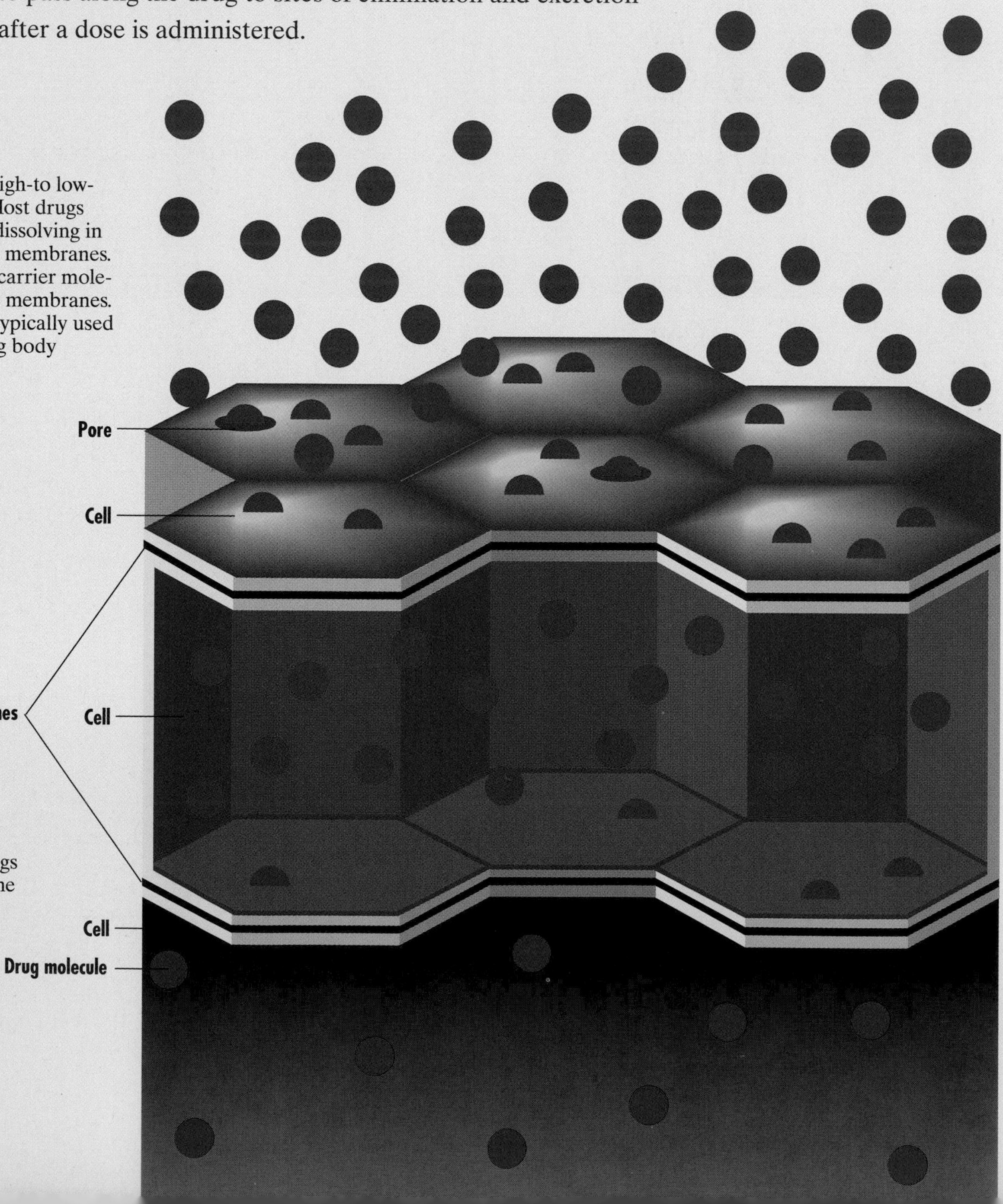

If the molecules are very small, drugs can move through openings (pores, channels) in the membranes.

Pore

Cell

Membranes

Cell

Cell

Drug molecule

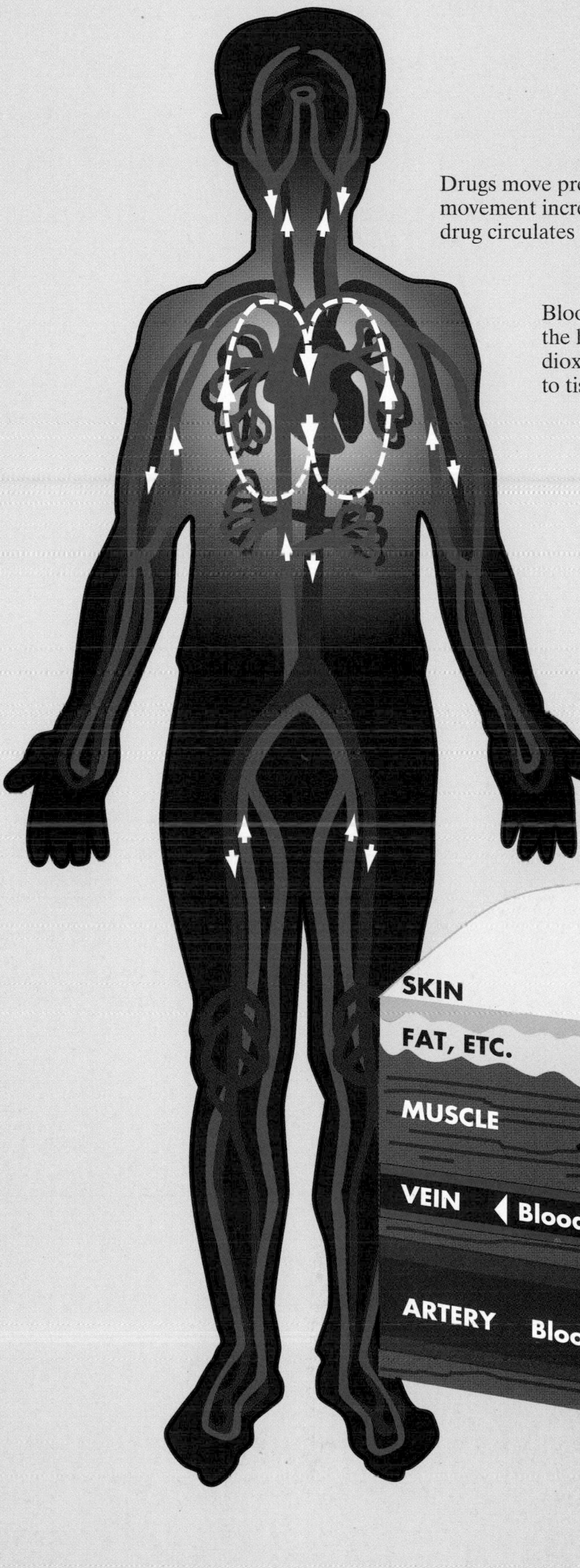

Drugs move predictably throughout the body and drug movement increases in speed and distance once the drug circulates in the bloodstream.

Blood moves from tissues to the heart via veins. It goes from the heart to the lungs to obtain oxygen and release carbon dioxide. Blood then goes back to the heart before returning to tissues via arteries, carrying the drug along with it.

Drugs can be taken orally or inhaled into the lungs or into the nose. They may also be injected through the skin into a layer of fat or muscle or into a vein (intravenously). Intravenous injection produces the most rapid effect.

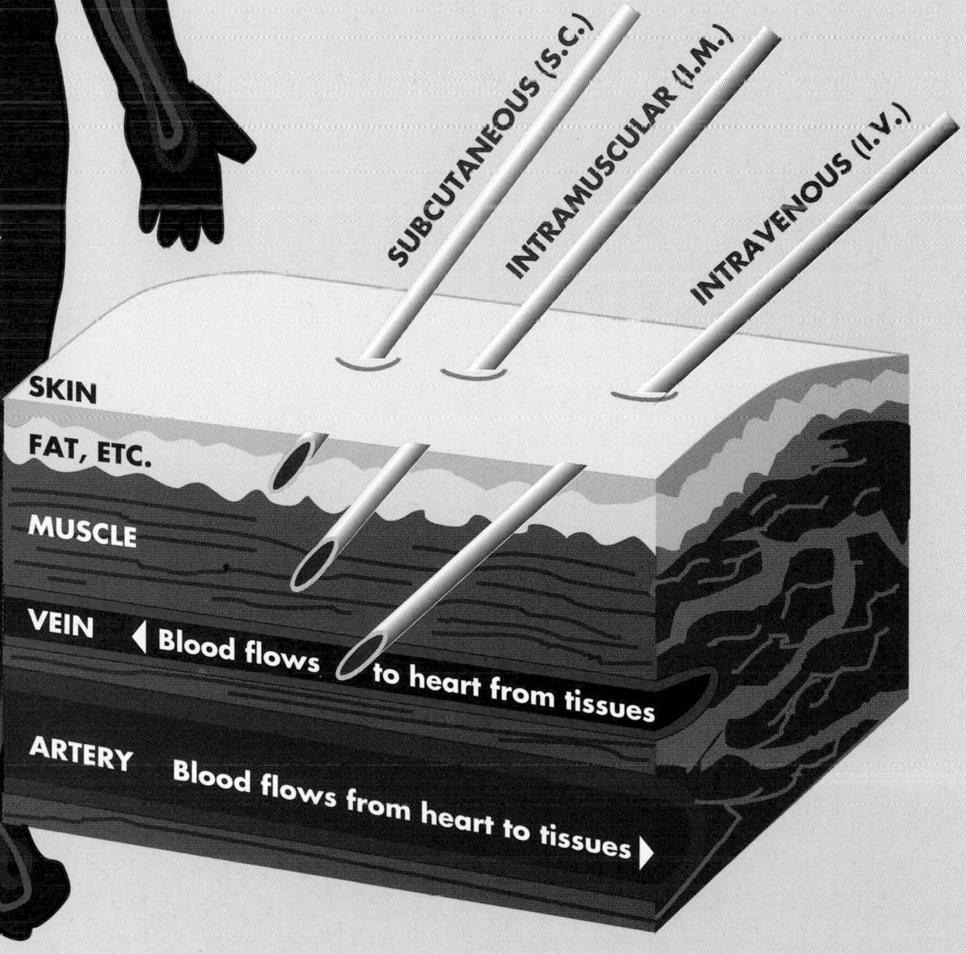

SUBCUTANEOUS (S.C.)

INTRAMUSCULAR (I.M.)

INTRAVENOUS (I.V.)

SKIN

FAT, ETC.

MUSCLE

VEIN ◀ Blood flows to heart from tissues

ARTERY Blood flows from heart to tissues ▶

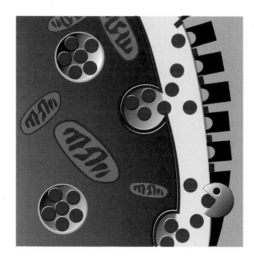

CHAPTER 3

How Drugs Interact with the Brain

THE DRUGS DISCUSSED in this book affect the brain. The brain is a major part of the body's central nervous system (CNS); the spinal cord is the other part. Body functions are controlled in localized areas of the brain, although an area of the brain may be involved in more than one function.

The brain is divided structurally into several main sections. The *brain stem* is the oldest and most primitive part of the brain. Control centers for essential body processes such as respiration occur in the brain stem. Between the brain stem and the uppermost part of the brain, the *cerebrum*, is the *diencephalon*, which has two main divisions. One is the *thalamus*, which functions as a central relay station for information going to and from the cerebrum. Signals that pass through the thalamus may be modified in the process. For example, this is where pain perception, muscle tone, and numerous other features can be adjusted. The *hypothalamus* is the second part of the diencephalon. It interacts with the rest of the CNS, synthesizes hormones, and regulates settings for basic body functions such as temperature and heart rate. The outer parts of the cerebrum are divided into lobes. Large overall body functions such as movement are localized within areas of these lobes. Beneath the lobes are additional structures, the basal nuclei. The basal nuclei are involved in control of movement.

The CNS contains hundreds of millions of neurons. Neurons are a special type of cell that carry information between the brain and other parts of the body.

Neurons send and receive information via chemical signals. These chemicals are called neurotransmitters. Some drugs resemble neurotransmitters. As a result, these drugs can either mimic or block the action of the neurotransmitter they resemble. Drugs that mimic these actions are called agonists and those that block action are called antagonists, or blockers.

Neurotransmitters are made within neurons and are released from the terminals, or ends, of a long thin projection, the axon. Incoming signals either stimulate or inhibit the neuron's membrane. If a neuron is stimulated to the point that its membrane reaches a threshhold, this produces an action potential. An *action potential* is a spikelike electrical signal that travels along the axon to the terminal. As a result, some vesicles fuse with the surface membrane and release neurotransmitters.

Vesicles are small sacs in the axon terminals that store neurotransmitters until a signal for release is issued by a neuron. The released neurotransmitter then acts on one or more additional cells to continue the communication process. The frequency of action potentials in the sending neuron controls the amount of neurotransmitter released in any time period; the intensity of effect that occurs on the receiving cell is directly related to the amount of neurotransmitter acting on it. The result of a communication sequence is a thought, perception, mood, movement, and so forth, with a variable intensity.

Many of the drugs discussed in this book resemble specific neurotransmitters and those drugs can interact with the neurotransmitter's receptors. This means the actions of drugs that resemble neurotransmitters can often be explained, and even predicted, by knowing where in the brain the neurotransmitter acts and what functions are controlled by that area.

The five following neurotransmitters will be referenced throughout this book: norepinephrine (NOR-eppa-neffrin); dopamine (DOPE-a-meen); serotonin (serro-TOE-nin); acetylcholine (a-set-il-KOH-leen); and gamma-aminobutyric (gamma-a-MEENO-b'yu-terik) acid, or GABA. Norepinephrine is found in structures of the reticular formation, especially the locus ceruleus. It also occurs in the hypothalamus and in the limbic system, thalamus, and projections of the frontal cortex. The cerebellum is also a site of norepinephrine. The effects of norepinephrine include alertness, focus, positive emotions, and analgesia, which is the suppression of the sensation of pain. Too little norepinephrine is involved in depression and also in the inability to focus attention; excess norepinephrine can result in impulsive behaviors and anxiety. Methamphetamine, or speed, mimics the effects of norepinephrine.

Dopamine is found at high levels in the limbic system. Euphoria is one of the effects of dopamine. Excess dopamine is associated with psychotic behavior, including hallucinations and paranoia. Too little dopamine in the basal ganglia is involved in the movement disorder known as Parkinson's disease. Cocaine mimics the effects of dopamine.

The areas of the brain that contain high levels of serotonin generally parallel those where norepinephrine is high as well. Serotonin is found in the reticular formation, limbic system structures, and the hypothalamus. Typically, serotonin is inhibitory to activity and behavior. A shortage of serotonin appears to be involved in mood, compulsive behavior, and in other inappropriate behaviors. Drugs related to LSD interact with serotonin receptors. These drugs cause stimulation or inhibition as a function of dose.

Acetylcholine is the neurotransmitter found in the terminals of peripheral motor neurons, the nerves that are associated with skeletal muscle and which allow voluntary movement. In the central nervous system (CNS), acetylcholine is found in the motor cortex and in an area known as the nucleus basalis, which is beneath the basal nuclei and thalamus. In Alzheimer's disease, there is a loss of acetylcholine and dependent structures. There is also a loss of associated functions, such as memory. Acetylcholine is also involved in arousal, learning, mood, and sleep. Scopolamine (sko-POLE-a-meen) is a long known and sometimes abused drug that prevents the actions of acetylcholine. It produces amnesic effects occurring through the block of cortex receptors. Nicotine mimics the effects of acetylcholine.

GABA is an inhibitory neurotransmitter that is found extensively throughout the brain. An excess of GABA in the basal nuclei may occur in Parkinson's disease. Alcohol and barbiturates mimic the effects of GABA.

How Nerve Cells Converse

The functions of the brain reflect the function of its unit structure, the neuron. This illustration shows the special structural features of a neuron. The synapse is a communications connection that exists between an axon terminal and the receptor site for another neuron.

Nerve cells, or *neurons*, communicate with each other (and with other types of cells outside the nervous system) through chemical signals, or neurotransmitters.

Axon

The release of a neurotransmitter is elicited by a brief (1–2 millisecond) electrical signal, or *action potential,* which usually starts at the junction of a neuron's cell body and its axon and travels unidirectionally to the axon's tip, or *terminal.*

Action potential

Neurotransmitter

Synapse

Receptor site

Positive and negative chemical charges exist inside and outside cells. However, the distribution of charges differs. The distribution difference results in an electrical signal across the cell membrane called the *membrane potential.* Neurotransmitters change the membrane potential by interacting with receptors that occur at several possible sites on neurons. Each neurotransmitter changes the potential in a predictable way: some stimulate (+) the neuron while others inhibit (–) it. More than one neurotransmitter may act on a neuron at one time. In this case, the membrane potential change is the sum, or net, effect from all of the neurotransmitters involved.

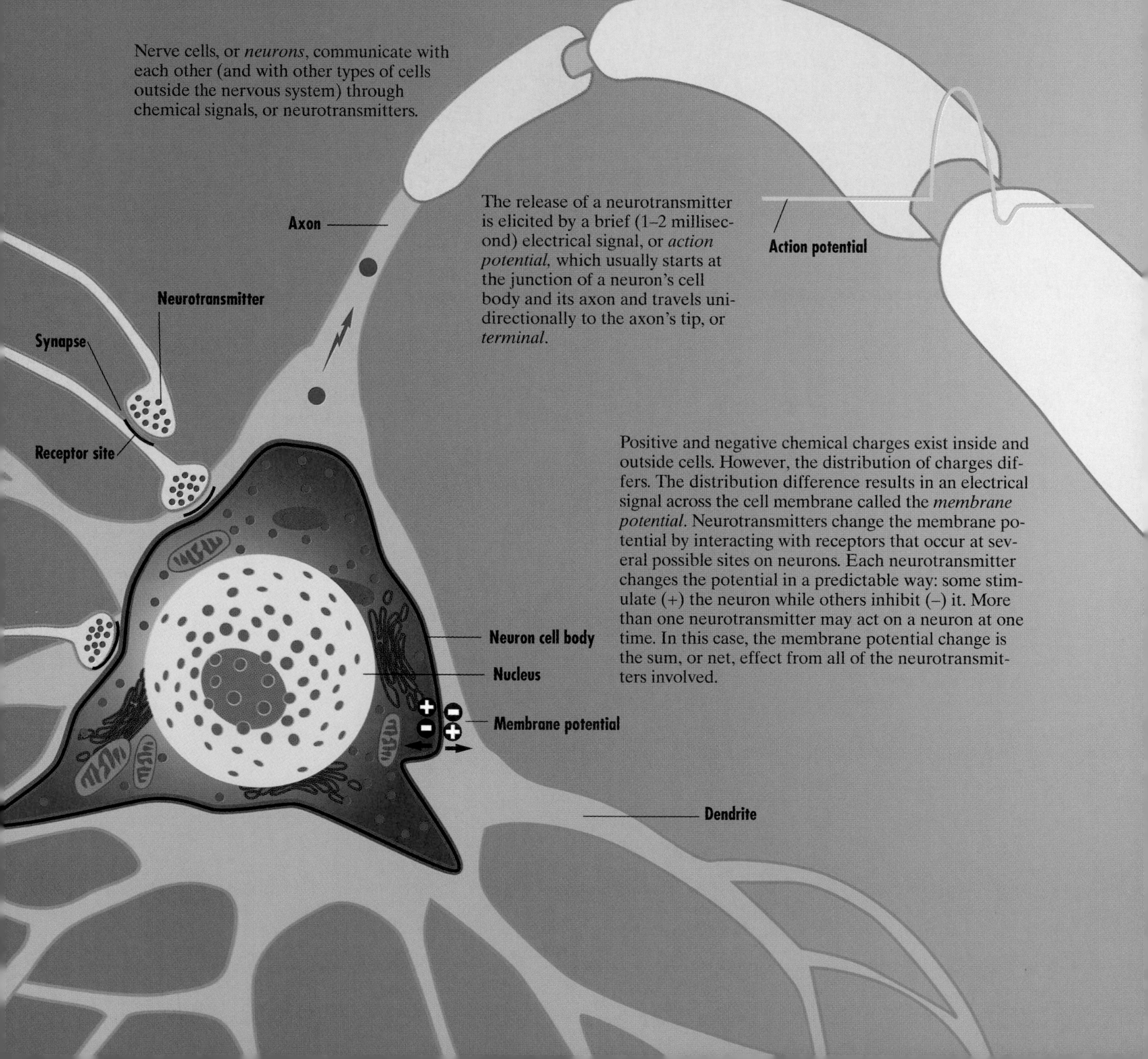

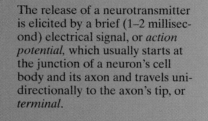

Neuron cell body

Nucleus

Membrane potential

Dendrite

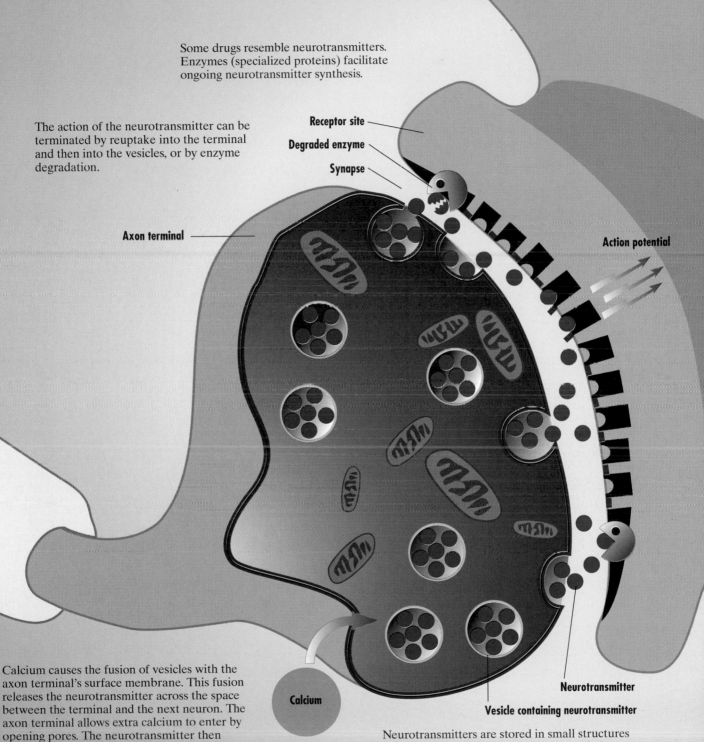

Some drugs resemble neurotransmitters. Enzymes (specialized proteins) facilitate ongoing neurotransmitter synthesis.

The action of the neurotransmitter can be terminated by reuptake into the terminal and then into the vesicles, or by enzyme degradation.

Receptor site

Degraded enzyme

Synapse

Axon terminal

Action potential

Calcium causes the fusion of vesicles with the axon terminal's surface membrane. This fusion releases the neurotransmitter across the space between the terminal and the next neuron. The axon terminal allows extra calcium to enter by opening pores. The neurotransmitter then combines with receptors for another neuron.

Calcium

Neurotransmitter

Vesicle containing neurotransmitter

Neurotransmitters are stored in small structures called vesicles. Neurotransmitters remain in these vesicles until an action potential occurs and reaches the axon terminal, causing the neuro-transmitters to be released.

Major Areas of the Brain

The brain can be described in several ways, using large structural features, systems, or functions as points of reference. Structures involved in some specific functions that are affected by the drugs discussed in later sections are shown on the opposite page.

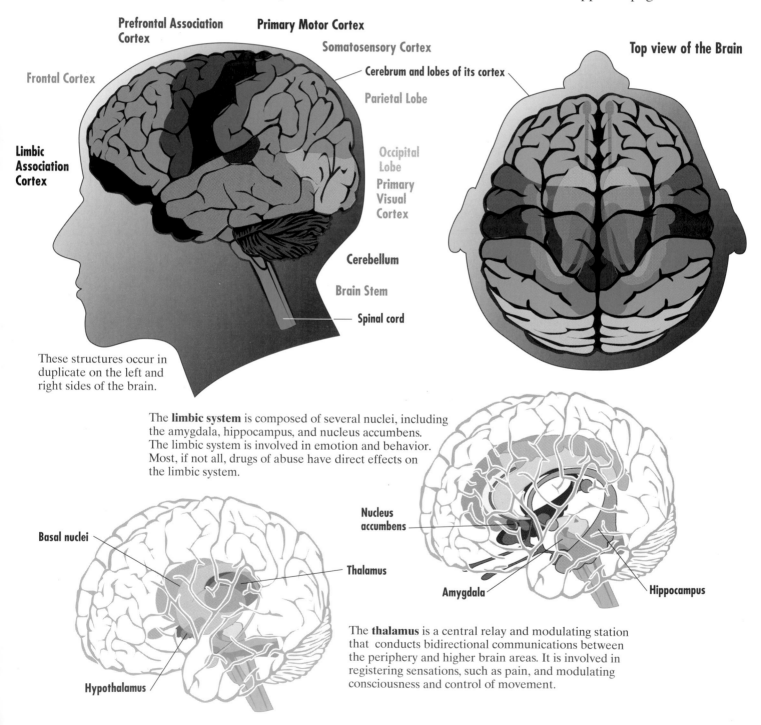

Prefrontal Association Cortex

Primary Motor Cortex

Somatosensory Cortex

Top view of the Brain

Frontal Cortex

Cerebrum and lobes of its cortex

Parietal Lobe

Occipital Lobe

Limbic Association Cortex

Primary Visual Cortex

Cerebellum

Brain Stem

Spinal cord

These structures occur in duplicate on the left and right sides of the brain.

The **limbic system** is composed of several nuclei, including the amygdala, hippocampus, and nucleus accumbens. The limbic system is involved in emotion and behavior. Most, if not all, drugs of abuse have direct effects on the limbic system.

Basal nuclei

Nucleus accumbens

Thalamus

Amygdala

Hippocampus

Hypothalamus

The **thalamus** is a central relay and modulating station that conducts bidirectional communications between the periphery and higher brain areas. It is involved in registering sensations, such as pain, and modulating consciousness and control of movement.

The **reticular formation** is the core of the brain stem. Signals from peripheral sensory fibers, especially pain signals, as well as signals from the eyes and ears, pass through the reticular formation. They may be modified in the reticular formation and then continue upward through the thalamus and on to areas of the cerebral cortex. The upward signals from the reticular formation modify the degree of alertness. Downward signals from the reticular formation modify pain signals at their level of entry in the spinal cord. The reticular formation also contains a sleep-inducing area.

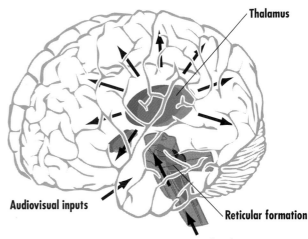

Thalamus

Audiovisual inputs

Reticular formation

Peripheral sensory inputs

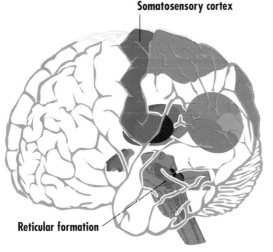

Somatosensory cortex

Reticular formation

These are some of the brain areas that are involved in sensation and perception.

The body sends sensory and perceptional information to the somatosensory cortex from the spinal cord through the reticular activating system and the thalamus. Opium derivatives, which are used for pain relief, alter pain sensation and awareness in the somatosensory cortex.

Sensory information from the eyes and ears is relayed to different areas of the cortex. Other types of sensory information are sent to additional cortical areas for integration and are then relayed to areas controlling voluntary movement, speech, and more. The neurotransmitters GABA and acetylcholine are released through the cortex. GABA is associated with alcohol and barbituates. Acetylcholine is associated with nicotine.

These are some of the brain areas that are involved in emotion, behavior, and motivation. Stimulation of these structures, most of which belong to the limbic system, can cause pleasure, aversion, anger, excitability, and aggression. The nucleus accumbens is associated with pleasure; the amygdala with aversion; the lateral hypothalamus with anger; and the middle hypothalamus with excitability and aggression. Limbic stimulation can also elicit motivation and locomotion.

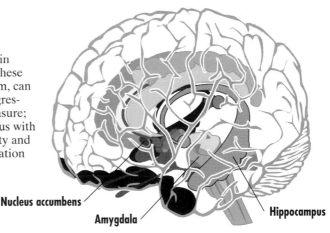

Nucleus accumbens

Amygdala

Hippocampus

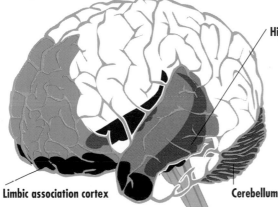

Hippocampus

Limbic association cortex

Cerebellum

These are some of the brain areas that are involved in memory. There are three different types of memory: short term, long term, and procedural. The hippocampus and the limbic association cortex handle short- and long-term memory. Procedural memory occurs for sequences of automatic movements. In order to routinely drive a car with a standard transmission, for example, you rely on procedural memory. Marijuana has direct effects on these structures. Procedural memory is associated with the cerebellum.

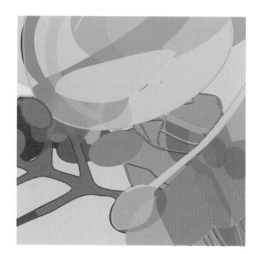

How the Reward Circuit Works

THE REWARD CIRCUIT is a final, common pathway in the brain that drugs follow. It ordinarily functions in providing humans a reason, or a reward such as intense pleasure, for carrying out various activities. Eating, sex, and nuturing are common examples of these types of activities. The reward circuit interacts directly or indirectly with many areas and systems in the brain, including those involved in alertness, emotions, memory, motivation, movement, equilibrium, and control of hormones.

Many of these interactions have significant consequences. For those that are associated with pleasure, the pleasure itself is remembered as a reward in association with the activity that caused it, and that memory provides motivation to experience the reward again. The reward circuit, like all circuits in the brain, functions through neurotransmitters, especially dopamine. In order for a drug of abuse to interact with the reward circuit, the only behavior required to produce a reward is the taking of the drug: The effects of the drug in the brain result in altered activity in the reward circuit, and the reward (pleasure, euphoria, altered performance) is experienced. Drugs of abuse as divergent in effects as cocaine and morphine have been shown to affect the brain's reward system.

Several types of experiments have been done to determine how the neurotransmitter dopamine interacts with the reward circuit. In one experiment, brain areas were manipulated and the resulting changes in behavior noted. It was found that removing an area of neurons involved in the circuit reduces or even obliterates reward-dependent behavior. It was also discovered that using a drug such as cocaine, which mimics the effects of the neurotransmitter dopamine, to stimulate the neurons could produce a reward without need of any other reward-dependent behavior. In yet other experiments, actual levels of dopamine in the reward circuit have been determined as a function of behavior or stimulation of a brain area, with and without the presence of drugs in the body.

How Drug Effects Reinforce Drug Taking

Using drugs of abuse frequently produces drug-seeking behavior. Many drugs of abuse, such as cocaine, can activate the reward circuit of the brain. The direct effects of a particular drug on the reward circuit are to produce sensations of pleasure, change performance, and so on. The indirect effects of a drug are related to a particular setting, place, or memory. These effects can initiate drug-seeking behavior, as well as reinforce it.

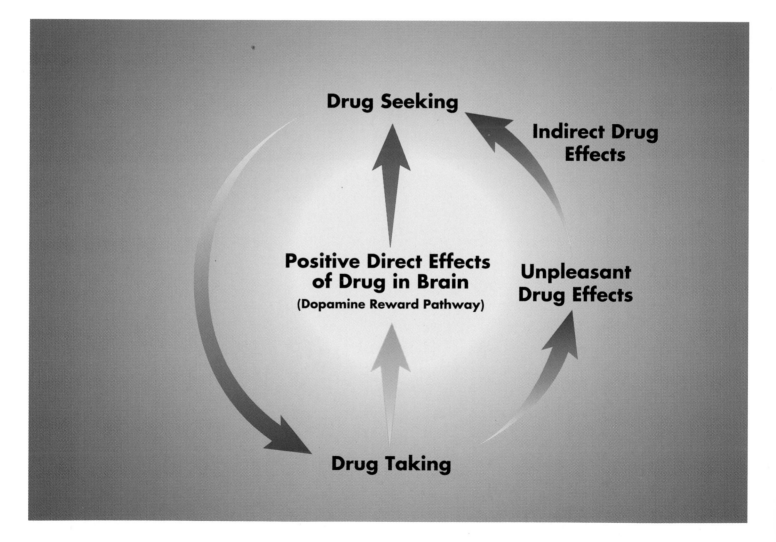

The central reward circuit goes from an area in the midbrain (ventral tegmental area) to a specific nucleus in the limbic system (nucleus accumbens), and from there to areas of the cerebral cortex and basal nuclei. The cell bodies of the dopamine neurons are located in the VTA, and their terminals are in the NA. Other neurotransmitters can modify the amount of dopamine released in the NA, or even modify the function of the neurons onto which dopamine is released.

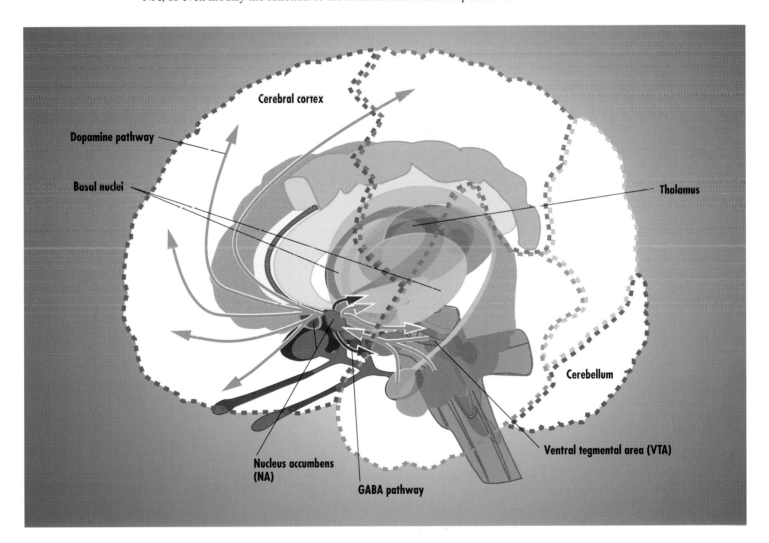

There may be two additional circuits involved in the common reward system for drugs. In particular, the circuits from the NA to an area of one of the basal nuclei and from the NA to an area below the limbic system. The function of both these circuits involves motor activity and the neurotransmitter GABA.

CHAPTER
5

How Drug Testing Works

EXTENSIVE, ACCURATE, AND sensitive screening and confirmatory analytic tests have been developed for drugs of abuse. The primary goal of drug testing is the improvement of job safety. These tests can be performed using biological samples of urine, saliva, blood, and even hair.

Comprehensive procedures and standards for testing have been described in detail in the Mandatory Guidelines for Federal Drug Testing Programs. Established in 1988, these guidelines list which drugs must or can be tested. They also list the types of tests that are acceptable; describe correct collection and handling of samples for testing; outline the certification requirements for labs that actually do the testing; and list the procedures to be followed when the test results are positive. The minimum testing requirements under the Mandatory Guidelines include marijuana and cocaine, although testing for opiates, amphetamines, phencyclidine (PCP), and others is authorized if there is sufficient reason (a workplace accident, for example).

Although numerous techniques for drug testing are widely available, the guidelines specifically require use of the best available technology by a certified laboratory. Strict sample-handling procedures are outlined from collection to testing to minimize the possibility of tampering, chemical instability, or physical loss of the sample. The screening test must be followed by a confirmatory test if the screen is positive. The confirmatory test must be done by a mass spectrometry method, which is explained in the illustration for this chapter. The result of this test must be positive for the overall test to be positive. If both tests are positive, the medical review officer, who is a physician familiar with substance abuse and its appropriate management, must review the results with the individual. One aim of this review is to identify other reasons for a positive result: Positive results cannot be forwarded to any administrative representative until this part of the review is complete.

How Drug Tests Work

Biological samples such as urine that are to be tested for drugs may require *conditioning*—treatment to concentrate the sample or to eliminate interfering substances that may cause a false positive or a false negative result.

Drug (Ⓓ) in biological sample

A standard, or authenic sample drug is always included during testing in order to assure the test is functioning properly and also to provide a basis for quantifying the unknown sample. Standards and unknown test samples are also run as *replicates*, duplicates of the same sample. They are created to avoid complete loss of the measurement if a tube breaks, for example.

Ⓓ

TEST READY
(Conditioned)

A *spectrophotometric test* causes a chemical reaction that produces a substance that absorbs a particular wavelength of light.

SPECTROPHOTOMETRY

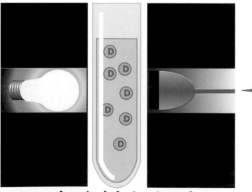

D (or a chemical derivative) changes the amount of light that goes through a sample in proportion to the amount of D (concentration).

CHROMATOGRAPHY

A *thin-layer chromatography test* separates the drug from other substances and identifies it by its movement on a solid-coated surface. The drug may also be passed through a column packed with a bead-form solid, which constitutes a *liquid chromatography test*. An additional spectrophotometric method may still be used to determine the amount of the drug present after its separation and identification.

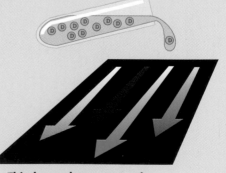

Thin layer chromatography

IMMUNOASSAY

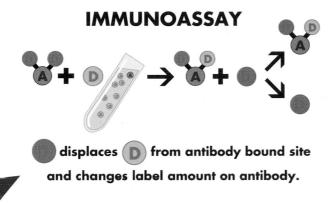

displaces **D** from antibody bound site and changes label amount on antibody.

An *immunoassay test* is based on an antibody that has been developed to detect a particular drug of abuse ans a specially prepared (labeled) drug. The drug of abuse that is present in the sample and the molecules of the drug with a detectable label, such as radioactivity, compete for antibody binding sites. The amount of the drug of abuse can be determined from the amount of the labeled drug that it displaces or frees from binding.

The *gas chromatography test* is similar to liquid chromatography, except that the separation occurs via movement in a solvent mixture that has been heated to a gaseous state.

The "gold standard" test method for drug identification is mass spectrometry. *Mass spectrometry* is almost always done with a sample that has already undergone some prior extensive separation—for example, by gas chromatography processing. The sample is fragmented and ionized and the ions are accelerated by an electrostatic field through a column surrounded by a magnetic field. (*Ions* are groups of atoms that contain positive and negative electrical charges.) The identity of the drug is determined from the pattern of ions.

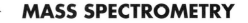

MASS SPECTROMETRY

Liquid (gas) chromatography

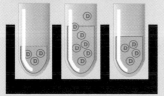

Test results

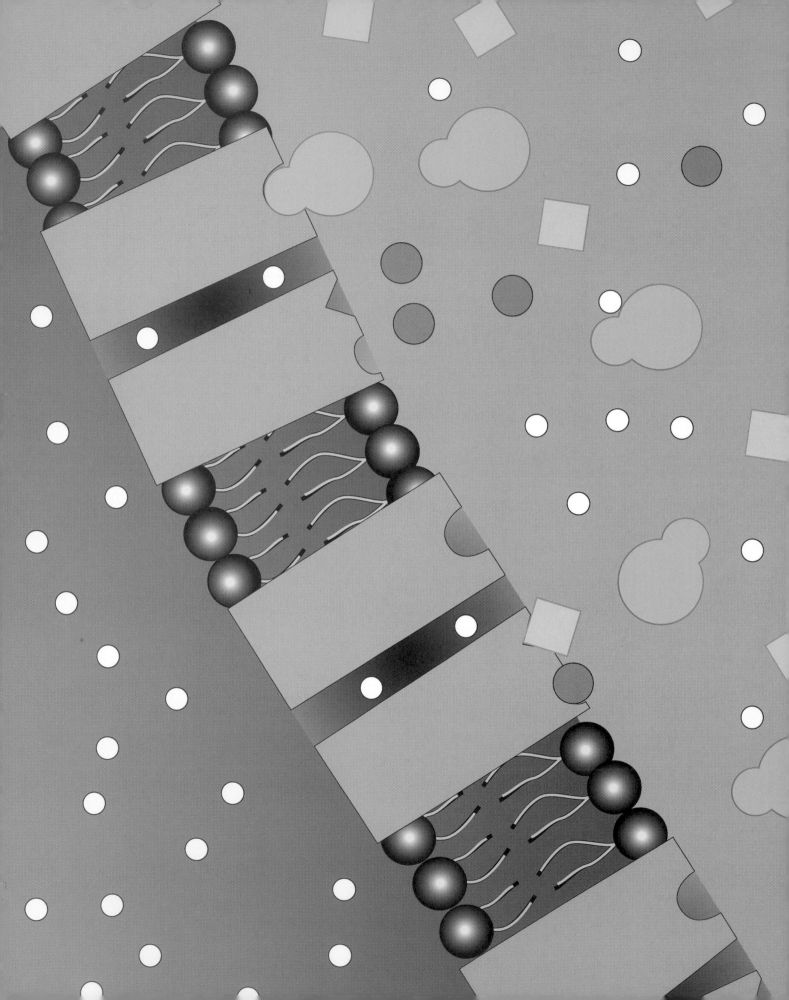

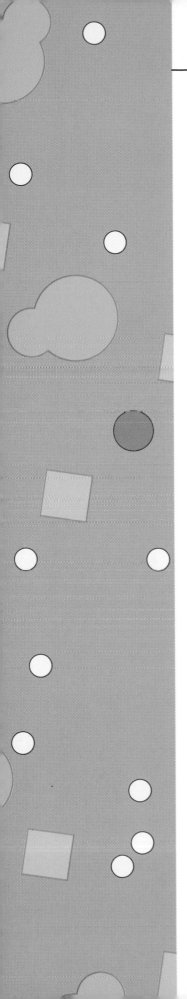

DEPRESSANT DRUGS

2

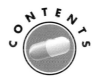

CONTENTS

THE DRUGS DISCUSSED in this section belong to several distinct, structurally unrelated chemical groups. However, these drugs have been grouped together to emphasize their similar effects.

Some dose of each of these drugs will produce central nervous system (CNS) depression, or decreased function. In fact, each of the drugs, taken at very high doses, is able to cause death, with the almost inevitable reason being respiratory failure as a result of CNS depression.

Specifically, the groups of depressants include alcohols (mainly ethanol), narcotics (opioids), inhalants (solvents and other volatile agents), barbiturates (sedatives), and benzodiazepines (anti-anxiety agents). *Disinhibition*, or overcoming inhibition, is the general mechanism by which these drugs may appear to cause stimulation.

Alcohol and the opioids (morphine and codeine) are among the oldest depressants. Alcohol is a yeast product. Humans long ago befriended the yeasts and learned to work with different varieties of them to produce numerous alcohol-containing beverages, such as beer.

The opioids are made from the opium poppy. Various parts of the opium poppy have been used for thousands of years, since the effects of their active ingredients were recognized. Opium latex, a white, milky fluid produced by the green seed pod, is still the source of morphine and codeine. It is also used for semisynthetic derivatives.

The inhalants as a group are diverse and difficult to place historically. Ethyl ether, which is the ether usually in reference, has been around since the 1500s, and was probably the earliest abused inhalant.

Barbiturates and benzodiazepines are synthetic creations of medicinal chemists; they date from the late 1800s and the mid 1900s, respectively.

Some effects of alcohol on the CNS may not involve specific receptors, in contrast to other depressant drugs. For example, there are specific sets of receptors for the narcotic drugs, such as morphine, and others for drugs like diazepam (Valium). The fact that diazepam and narcotics act on different receptors to cause the same general effect, that is, CNS depression, compounds their effects. Taking combinations of depressant drugs is extremely risky for this reason. Depressant drug interactions account for numerous accidental deaths by overdose.

Alcohol and some of the inhalants have unique detrimental effects on the body, even the CNS, subsequent to chronic use. Some of these effects occur because of the high lipid solubility that characterizes alcohol and some inhalants. A high lipid, or fat, solubility facilitates the movement and distribution of drugs in the body. In the case of alcohol and the inhalants, it probably also facilitates nonreceptor effects on cell membranes. These nonreceptor membrane effects can ultimately destroy some types of cells.

The metabolism of alcohol and/or its effects on cellular metabolism cause long-term adverse effects on organs such as the liver and the heart. Liver damage is one well-known potential consequence of chronic alcohol abuse that is related to liver alcohol metabolism. Liver damage may also be caused by some of the inhalants that are metabolized by the liver.

Somewhat less familiar, but of clear health concern, is the detrimental effect of alcohol and certain inhalants on the heart. Chronic alcohol abuse can cause a cardio-myopathy (weakening and dysfunction of heart muscle) that can be fatal. Certain inhalants also affect the heart, but more characteristically produce acute disturbances of the heartbeat rather than long-term damage.

Both alcohol and the inhalants can cause the brain to atrophy, or decrease in size. Atrophy of the brain is associated with decreases in functions such as memory and cognition, for example.

An important feature that appears to be shared by all depressants is an ability to activate the reward circuit within the brain. Most of the drugs appear to influence the circuit, at least in part, by enhancing the effect of the neurotransmitter GABA (gamma aminobutyric acid). GABA is an inhibitory neurotransmitter—it decreases the excitability of neurons on which receptors for GABA are located.

The detailed effects and mechanisms of action for each class of depressant are described in the following chapters.

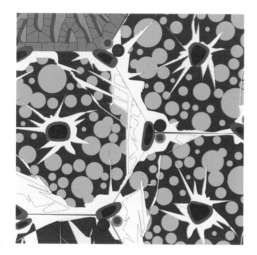

How Alcohol Works

ALCOHOL MAY BE humankind's oldest drug. It is surely our oldest abused drug. Beer-making, using cultivated barley, and wine-making, from vineyard grapes, were firmly established by about 3500–4000 B.C. Alcohol-containing beverages may have been deliberately produced as early as 6000–8000 B.C.

Alcohol, like other drugs that are abused, reinforces its own consumption through activation of the brain's reward circuit. Alcohol causes numerous acute effects, such as inebriation, most of which result from depression of the central nervous system (CNS). The acute effects of alcohol have significant consequences, including judgment problems.

Repeated consumption of alcohol can induce tolerance, which means the amount necessary to produce the desired effect must be progressively increased. Repeated high-level consumption over long periods of time also adds a host of chronic effects to the acute ones, including physical dependence, damage to organs (in particular the stomach, liver, and brain), increased blood pressure, and aggravation of other medical problems.

Methanol (wood alcohol), ethylene glycol (antifreeze), and other alcohols are sometimes consumed by accident or when alcohol is unavailable. Methanol causes blindness and ethylene glycol causes severe kidney damage and failure. Ironically, alcohol can be useful in the treatment of poisoning by both. Methanol and ethylene glycol are metabolized by the same enzymes that metabolize alcohol. The enzymes will metabolize the alcohol first even if the other compounds are present. Since the substances required to metabolize alcohol and ethylene glycol are responsible for their damage, occupying the enzymes with alcohol prevents metabolism and formation of the damaging products. The compounds are then handled by alternative systems and are excreted without causing as much harm.

Certain health benefits are associated with imbibing alcohol. Moderate consumption can result in a small reduction in blood lipid, or fat, levels and a modest shift in favor of "good" cholesterol. Both of these may reduce the risk of atherosclerosis, heart attacks, and strokes. These beneficial changes in blood lipids can also be obtained by other means, such as moderate routine exercise, which lacks the other potential effects of alcohol.

How the Acute Effects of Alcohol Occur

Alcohol depresses, or reduces the functionality of, the brain as a function of its concentration in blood (see below). The concentration of alcohol in blood is usually given as *% alcohol*. This percentage refers to the number of grams (a gram is about ⅟₃₀ of an ounce) of alcohol in 100 milliliters (ml) (about ⅓ cup) of blood. Most states have a legal limit of 0.1%, but some have lowered the limit to 0.08% in recognition of the fact that judgment and coordination are impaired at levels lower than 0.1%.

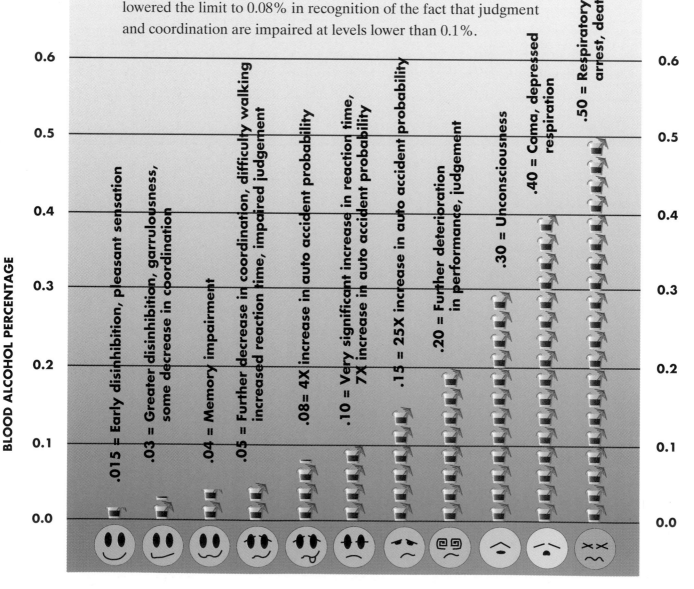

BLOOD ALCOHOL PERCENTAGE

.015 = Early disinhibition, pleasant sensation

.03 = Greater disinhibition, garrulousness, some decrease in coordination

.04 = Memory impairment

.05 = Further decrease in coordination, difficulty walking increased reaction time, impaired judgement

.08 = 4X increase in auto accident probability

.10 = Very significant increase in reaction time, 7X increase in auto accident probability

.15 = 25X increase in auto accident probability

.20 = Further deterioration in performance, judgement

.30 = Unconsciousness

.40 = Coma, depressed respiration

.50 = Respiratory arrest, death

EFFECTS

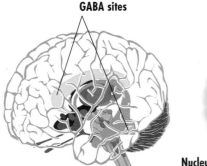

GABA sites

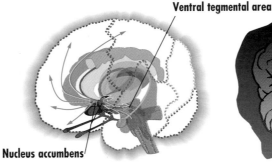

Ventral tegmental area

Nucleus accumbens

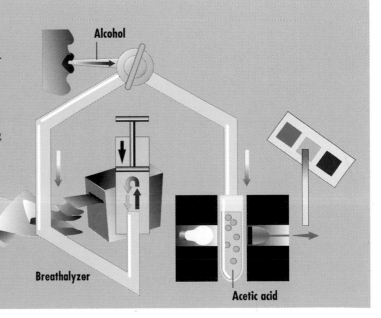

Blood-alcohol levels that will result from consuming certain amounts of alcohol cannot be easily predicted. This is due to the large number of factors that influence absorption rate, including food in the stomach, the dilution and total volume of alcohol, liver function status, gender, and metabolism after alcohol consumption. Alcohol is metabolized at a fixed rate that is proportional to body weight. On average, approximately 10 ml pure alcohol per hour, or about an ounce in 3 hours, is metabolized. A rule of thumb for allowing blood alcohol to return to legal limits is to allow an hour for every one or two drinks consumed. The amount of alcohol needed to produce various intoxication levels in an average consumer are shown in this chart.

The chemical properties of alcohol allow it to be easily absorbed from the stomach into the bloodstream. From blood, it likewise enters the brain without restriction. The same chemical properties of alcohol allow it to enter and change the properties of cell membranes. Neurons that are exposed to alcohol may not conduct action potentials as frequently or as rapidly as normal. This accounts for some of alcohol's widespread depressant effects on the brain. Alcohol activates the brain's reward circuit, most likely by enhancing the inhibitory actions of the neurotransmitter GABA (gamma-aminobutyric acid) in one part of the circuit, the ventral tegmental area (VTA). GABA is an inhibitory neurotransmitter that is found extensively throughout the brain. Alcohol also appears to act on a subset of GABA receptors. Antagonists at that site limit alcohol intake and also reverse some effects of alcohol, suggesting a possible use in the treatment of inebriation.

Levels of alcohol in the lungs are related to those in blood. In alcohol breath tests, a sample of expired air is collected in a closed chamber through tubing connected to a mouthpiece. In instruments designed for immediate processing, part of the sample is then flushed into a solution, across an electrode, or through an infrared photocell. In instruments that use a solution, alcohol is converted to acetic acid; the color of the solution and its absorption of colored light changes in direct proportion to the amount of acetic acid. In instruments using an electrode for detection, a change in the electrode's potential due to alcohol on the electrode is detected. In an infrared instrument, a change in infrared light absorption is measured. There are color-coded result indicators (green-yellow-red, for pass-questionable-fail) on some instruments, while others have a digital output. Most instruments also produce some type of printed output for records purposes.

Alcohol

Breathalyzer

Acetic acid

The Chronic Effects of Alcohol

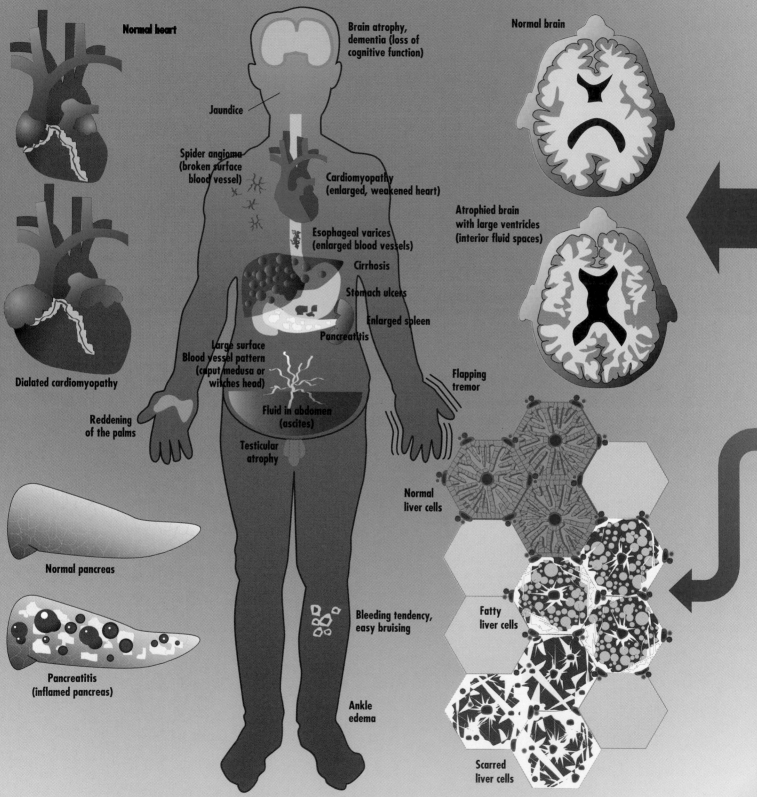

Normal heart

Brain atrophy, dementia (loss of cognitive function)

Normal brain

Jaundice

Spider angioma (broken surface blood vessel)

Cardiomyopathy (enlarged, weakened heart)

Atrophied brain with large ventricles (interior fluid spaces)

Esophageal varices (enlarged blood vessels)

Cirrhosis

Stomach ulcers

Enlarged spleen

Pancreatitis

Dialated cardiomyopathy

Large surface Blood vessel pattern (caput medusa or witches head)

Flapping tremor

Reddening of the palms

Fluid in abdomen (ascites)

Testicular atrophy

Normal liver cells

Normal pancreas

Bleeding tendency, easy bruising

Fatty liver cells

Pancreatitis (inflamed pancreas)

Ankle edema

Scarred liver cells

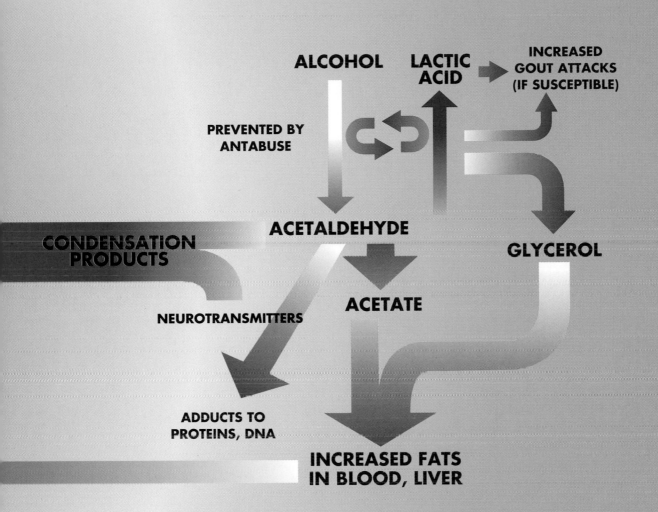

ALCOHOL · LACTIC ACID · INCREASED GOUT ATTACKS (IF SUSCEPTIBLE)

PREVENTED BY ANTABUSE

ACETALDEHYDE

CONDENSATION PRODUCTS

GLYCEROL

NEUROTRANSMITTERS

ACETATE

ADDUCTS TO PROTEINS, DNA

INCREASED FATS IN BLOOD, LIVER

Chronic alcohol abuse over a period of years damages organ systems throughout the body, including the brain. After alcohol is consumed, it is converted to acetaldehyde. The conversion of alcohol to acetaldehyde leads to the production of lactic acid. An excess of lactic acid in the body can increase symptoms of gout in suscepitble individuals. Gout is an inherited metabolic disorder. Acetaldehyde reacts with neurotransmitters to form condensation products. High acetaldehyde levels are found in those who ingest large amounts of alcohol repetitively as well as in those who cannot convert it at a normal rate. Increased alcohol intake and metabolism also trigger an increase in lipids, or fats, in the blood and in the liver. Proteins and DNA may be damaged when excess acetaldehyde reacts with them: DNA is the genetic material of cells; proteins provide structure and numerous cellular functions.

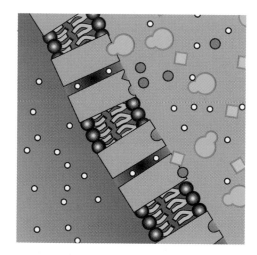

How Downers Work

DOWNERS ARE CENTRAL nervous system (CNS) depressants that can reduce anxiety and induce sleep or even anesthesia. Barbiturates and benzodiazepines are the two main types of downers. Neither type is based on a natural product; both contain synthetic chemicals. The first barbiturate was synthesized in the late 1800s by German chemist Alfred von Baeyer. The first compound, diethylbarbituric acid, was derived from barbituric acid.

The unpredictable effects and duration of early derivatives of barbituric acid have subsequently been improved. One feature remains common to all barbiturates: There is only a slight difference between a dose that produces sedation and a dose that may cause death. Accidental death by overdose, particularly if alcohol is also used, is one concern associated with the use of barbiturates; suicide is another.

Phenobarbital, or Luminal, is a long-acting barbiturate that is effective in treating grand mal epilepsy. As a result of its long-lasting effects, phenobarbital may produce a hangover when the consumer wakes up because the effects are still acting. Barbiturates synthesized since phenobarbital have faster onset times and shorter durations, thus less effect and less of a hangover. Shorter-acting barbiturates include buta-, pento-, hexa-, and secobarbital.

Benzodiazepines are used more widely than barbiturates. The first benzodiazepine compound, chlordiazepoxide (Librium) was discovered accidentally in the early 1960s. Numerous relatives are in current clinical use, with familiar examples being diazepam (Valium) and triazolam (Halcion). Benzodiazepines and barbituiates can induce tolerance by increasing metabolism and causing cellular adaptations, and cause withdrawal symptoms. Barbituate withdrawal resembles alcohol withdrawal and can be severe, even life-threatening.

In contrast to the barbiturates, the most outstanding feature of the benzodiazepines is safety: There is a very large difference between an anxiety-reducing, sleep-inducing, or muscle-relaxing dose and a lethal dose, so much so that there is little possibility of accidental or deliberate death from these drugs used alone. However, using alcohol with benzodiazepines changes the safety picture. Benzodiazepines are fat soluble and are frequently metabolozed to additional compounds. These properties increase the duration of action and probability of hangover.

How Downers Cause CNS Depression

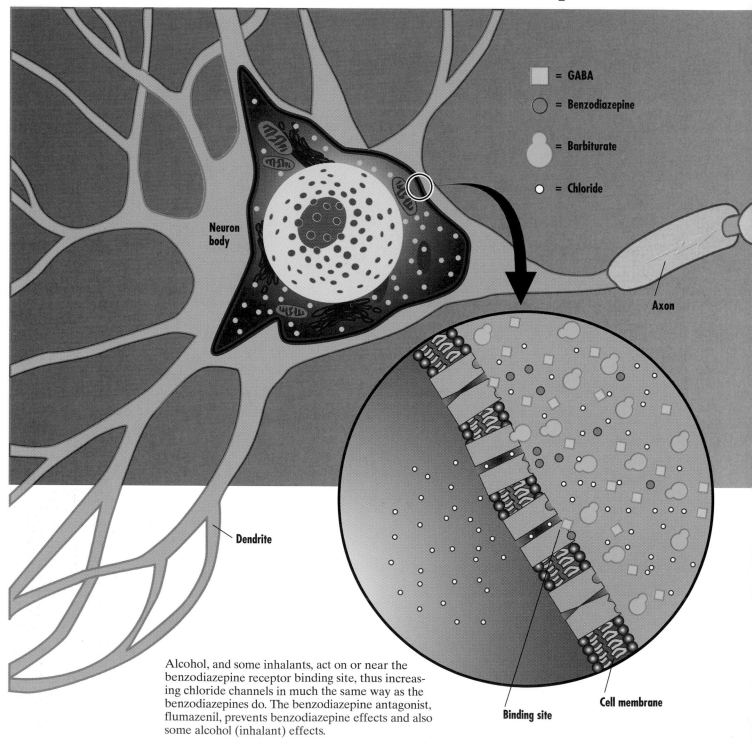

■ = GABA

◯ = Benzodiazepine

◯ = Barbiturate

○ = Chloride

Neuron body

Axon

Dendrite

Binding site

Cell membrane

Alcohol, and some inhalants, act on or near the benzodiazepine receptor binding site, thus increasing chloride channels in much the same way as the benzodiazepines do. The benzodiazepine antagonist, flumazenil, prevents benzodiazepine effects and also some alcohol (inhalant) effects.

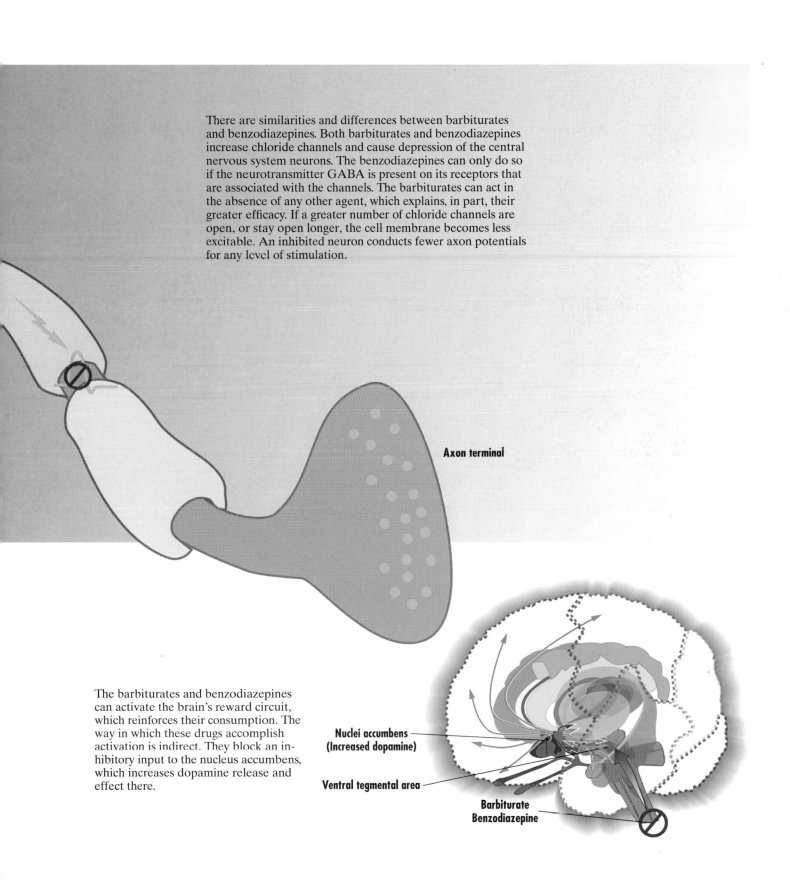

There are similarities and differences between barbiturates and benzodiazepines. Both barbiturates and benzodiazepines increase chloride channels and cause depression of the central nervous system neurons. The benzodiazepines can only do so if the neurotransmitter GABA is present on its receptors that are associated with the channels. The barbiturates can act in the absence of any other agent, which explains, in part, their greater efficacy. If a greater number of chloride channels are open, or stay open longer, the cell membrane becomes less excitable. An inhibited neuron conducts fewer axon potentials for any level of stimulation.

Axon terminal

The barbiturates and benzodiazepines can activate the brain's reward circuit, which reinforces their consumption. The way in which these drugs accomplish activation is indirect. They block an inhibitory input to the nucleus accumbens, which increases dopamine release and effect there.

Nuclei accumbens (Increased dopamine)

Ventral tegmental area

Barbiturate Benzodiazepine

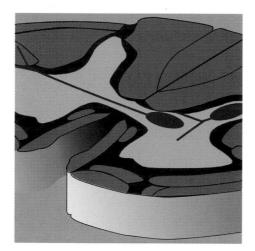

CHAPTER 8

How Narcotics Work

NARCOTICS ARE ALSO called opiates or opioids. Other drugs, particularly cocaine, are frequently and incorrectly called narcotics. Narcotics generally *depress*, or decrease the activity of, the central nervous system (CNS). Cocaine is a stimulant and will be discussed in a later section that deals with drugs in that category.

Narcotics include opium, the crude preparation from opium poppy juices, or latex; morphine and codeine, opium's main active principles; some semisynthetic and synthetic chemicals such as heroin and fentanyl; and also some peptides (small proteins) found in the brain itself.

Analgesia, or pain relief, and euphoria, an intense sense of pleasure and well-being, are two effects of narcotics. Respiratory depression accompanies both effects and is the cause of death due to overdose. The search for more effective narcotics has resulted in new, very potent opium derivatives such as fentanyl. Fentanyl is used medically as an analgesic. Unfortunately, it is also prized by abusers, who refer to it as China White.

Active drugs occur in all parts of the opium poppy. The term *opium* comes from the Greek for sap, indicating the juice, or latex, that can be collected from the green seed pods: The content of active principles in the latex is as high as 10%. The drug group name, *narcotics*, derives from a Greek term for stupor, a state resembling the deep sleep that can be induced by the narcotics. Opium has been used for thousands of years, perhaps as early as the fifteenth century B.C. in Egypt. Preparations and uses are described in several ancient documents. For example, a wine-opium combination for presurgical medication is described in a 3000 B.C. Chinese summary of considerably older practices.

Narcotics were introduced to the United States in the late 1800s by Chinese workers, who ate and smoked opium. Opium poppies were not introduced to Mexico and Central and South America (now major sites of cultivation for illicit world markets) until World War II. Morphine shortages during World War II led German chemists to synthesis of methadone as a substitute. Methadone is very long-acting and prevents euphoria in tolerant users. Because of this, it is a mainstay of detoxification and maintenance treatment programs.

Abuse is a recent problem in the history of narcotics. Until the seventeenth century, only crude and weak preparations were available, societal and medical norms regulated their use, and the drugs were taken orally. The introduction of smoking, administration by injection, the isolation of morphine, and the synthesis of heroin (so-called by its German developers because users felt heroic) all increased abuse probability. Drug dependence was not really understood as a physiologic and medical problem until the end of the nineteenth century, even though a written description of withdrawal symptoms dates from nearly 150 years earlier.

Concern about the problems of narcotics abuse and dependence intensified worldwide after the turn of this century with the introduction of heroin. Heroin is a semi-synthetic derivative of morphine that is ten times more potent than morphine and is able to enter the brain much more rapidly. This explains, in part, heroin's very high abuse liability.

Narcotic effects result from drug interaction with specific receptors in several areas of the CNS, including the reward circuit and the spinal cord. The brain contains the opioid neurotransmitters, which are the peptides known as endorphins and enkephalins. The latter are associated with runner's high and the modulation of individual pain tolerance.

Chronic use of narcotics can produce significant tolerance and dependence in the user, and also in a fetus carried by a user. A tolerant user may require 50–100 times the initial dose to provide a brief high. Sudden cessation of use in a tolerant user can cause intense and uncomfortable but not life-threatening withdrawal effects. Withdrawal symptoms are not as intense as those of alcohol or barbituates.

Symptoms associated with withdrawal include irritability, nausea and vomiting, insomnia, and gooseflesh. The term "gooseflesh" is the basis for describing sudden withdrawal as going "cold turkey." Tremors and twitching movements, particularly of the feet, occur and are the basis for another description of withdrawal, namely, kicking the habit. On average, withdrawal symptoms diminish 7–10 days after the last drug use.

How Narcotics Produce Effects

Specific receptors mediate narcotic effects. There are several types of receptors, denoted by the Greek letters mu (μ), kappa (κ), sigma (σ), and delta (δ). Mu and kappa receptors account for the majority of CNS effects that are discussed here. Sigma receptors, which can also be affected by the hallucinogen phencyclidine (PCP), account for some unwanted effects such as dysphoria, the opposite of euphoria, and hallucinations.

1 Mu receptors mediate the euphoric effects of narcotics in the reward circuit. They also mediate analgesia, as well as respiratory depression and some of the constipation that is associated with narcotic use. Additional narcotic effects associated with these receptors include excessive sweating, nausea (with initial vomiting which is later supressed), and cough suppression.

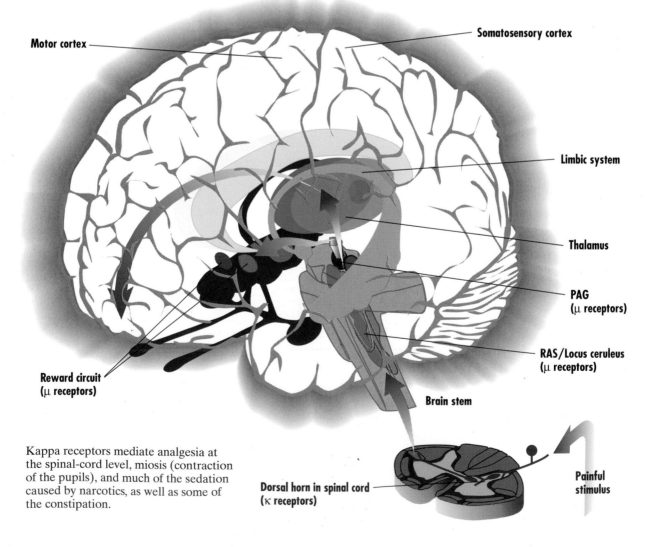

Motor cortex

Somatosensory cortex

Limbic system

Thalamus

PAG
(μ receptors)

RAS/Locus ceruleus
(μ receptors)

Reward circuit
(μ receptors)

Brain stem

Painful stimulus

Dorsal horn in spinal cord
(κ receptors)

Kappa receptors mediate analgesia at the spinal-cord level, miosis (contraction of the pupils), and much of the sedation caused by narcotics, as well as some of the constipation.

2 The energy storage compound ATP (adenosine triphosphate) is used to accomplish various cell functions. Tolerance develops in part because cells adapt to the narcotics. Narcotics function as first messengers that acutely inhibit the enzyme adenylate cyclase and decrease the second messenger cAMP, which is used to send signals between cells. Narcotics, as well as alcohol, also acutely limit calcium entry, which plays a role in sending signals. With chronic use, cellular cAMP and calcium adapt to the narcotic and return to normal levels as a result of increases in enzyme and calcium channels. Stopping drug use in a tolerant user causes withdrawal symptoms that reflect stimulation of previously depressed neurons.

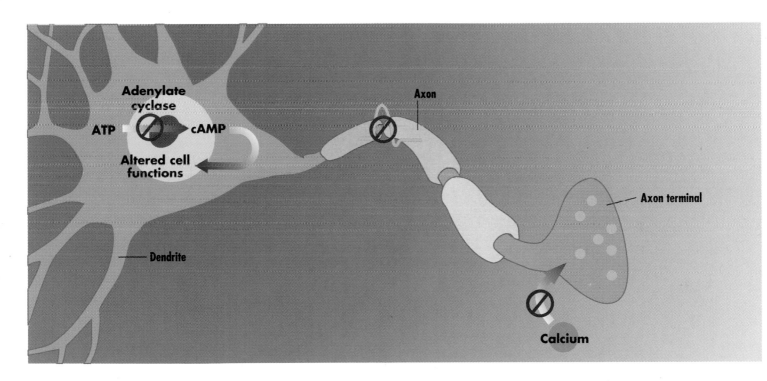

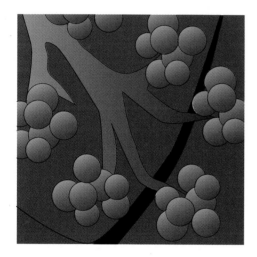

How Inhalants Work

THE BODY CAN absorb chemicals and drugs through the lungs by inhalation. This route of administration has been in use for a long time.

The strongest connection among the inhalants is their common route of use. However, most inhalants are central nervous system depressants with acute effects very similar to those of alcohol. In fact, many inhalant users simultaneously use other drugs, particularly alcohol. Importantly, the combined depressant effects of inhalants and alcohol can cause unexpected death.

The mechanism of depression may occur, in part, by increasing neuron chloride channels in the same way that alcohol increases them. As for alcohol, drugs that block the binding site where alcohol or inhalants act also block some inhalant effects. The long-term effects of inhalants differ among the various compounds, but a common property among many is neurotoxicity, or damage to nerves. Prolonged use of the neurotoxic agents can cause irreversible damage to peripheral and/or central nerves.

A volatile substance is one that converts readily to a vapor or gas, which are forms that are suitable for inhalation. Ironically, the development of inhalants is actually based on alcohol, which is not very volatile. Ethyl ether was synthesized from alcohol in the early 1500s. Ether shares many of alcohol's characteristics, such as ability to move easily through cell membranes, but unlike alcohol, it is very volatile. Ether was initially drunk rather than inhaled. It was used primarily by those who could not afford the newly available, expensive distilled alcoholic beverages. It quickly gained popularity.

The widespread recreational use of ether in so-called "ether frolics" gained the attention of medical practitioners by the mid-1800s. At that time there was no effective general anesthetic. Ether's potential as an anesthetic was recognized and it was soon in extensive use, especially during the Civil War. Abuse of other inhalants, such as chloroform and nitrous oxide, or laughing gas, has also led to medical use. Nitrous oxide is still used today.

Numerous volatile chemicals with very diverse structures have been produced that are used in medicine and industry and also by individuals. The list includes anesthetic agents, solvents, fuels, propellants, and more. A high-pressure solvent in an aerosol can is an example of a propellant. As the list continues to grow, so do opportunities for exposure and abuse. For example, some types of work can't be done without exposure to chemicals that can be abused as inhalants. One of the earliest reports of worksite abuse of an industrial solvent concerned young men inhaling trichloroethylene vapors at a British airplane repair facility in 1940. This report led to the short-lived use of trichloroethylene as an anesthetic. Use was later discontinued due to its neurotoxicity. Reports of gasoline inhalation and glue sniffing followed.

The acute symptoms of inhalant abuse are initial disinhibition, which may appear to be excitation, followed by incoordination, dizziness, disorientation, then muscle weakness, sometimes hallucinations, and eventually coma and death. Death can also occur early and rapidly with some inhalants due to disturbances of heart rhythm: This is called the Sudden Sniffing Death (SSD) syndrome. Heart effects are more likely if adrenalin levels are increased by running, excitation, or fear, for example. Fluorocarbons, available now mainly in fire extinguishers and certain anesthetic gases, are the main agents that can cause SSD. Death by suffocation can occur if an inhalant is breathed from a closed container. Inhalant vapor displaces the oxygen in the container and in the lungs. The lack of oxygen is not detected by the brain during intoxication due to the increasing depressant effects of the inhalant. Permanent brain damage can occur if the user survives.

Nitrites, such as amyl nitrite (poppers), are unusual among the inhalants because they do not depress the CNS. Rather, they relax blood vessels and decrease blood pressure, causing light-headedness and dizziness. While the latter may be perceived as a "high" by some, the main reason given for nitrite use is their purported enhancement of sexual pleasure.

How Inhalants Produce Effects

The chronic effects of inhalants vary by agent. Tolerance can occur for most: With time, increasing amounts must be used to produce effects. Withdrawal symptoms have been reported and are similar to those of alcohol. Some agents—for example, the solvent toluene—are very toxic to nerves.

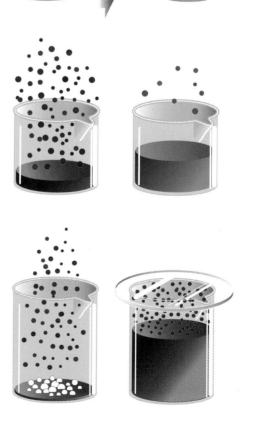

To be effective by inhalation, a substance must be gaseous to begin with or it must be *volatile*—able to convert from a liquid form to a vapor or gas.

A very volatile substance converts quickly, while a less volatile substance takes longer to convert.

The entire amount of a volatile liquid will evaporate if left open to air. Only a fraction vaporizes in a closed container, since a vapor pressure develops and limits further conversion.

One mechanism of toxicity is destruction of the insulating myelin around the nerve's axon fiber. This can cause damage to nerves outside the brain that are involved in sensation and/or motor function. Neurons within the brain can also be damaged in the same way as those in the periphery; myelin damage is independent of, and adds to, damage due to oxygen deprivation. A damaged neuron may not be able to transmit action potentials normally.

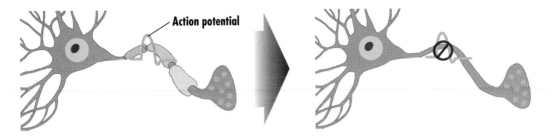

Action potential

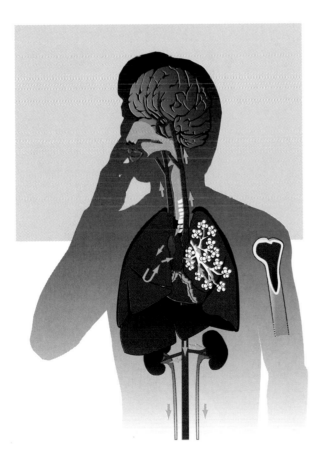

Inhalants may reduce the flow of oxygen to the brain, which can kill brain cells.

Once an inhalant enters the lungs, it then goes into the bloodstream. The chemicals in the blood reach the brain within seconds.

The abuse of some inhalants can cause bone marrow to become damaged. This may cause an insufficient production of red blood cells. Constant fatigue is a symptom of this condition.

Chronic contact with some inhalants may damage the kidneys and liver and reduce their function. If this happens, the body is less able to rid itself of toxins or usual by-products of metabolism (perhaps even the inhalant itself).

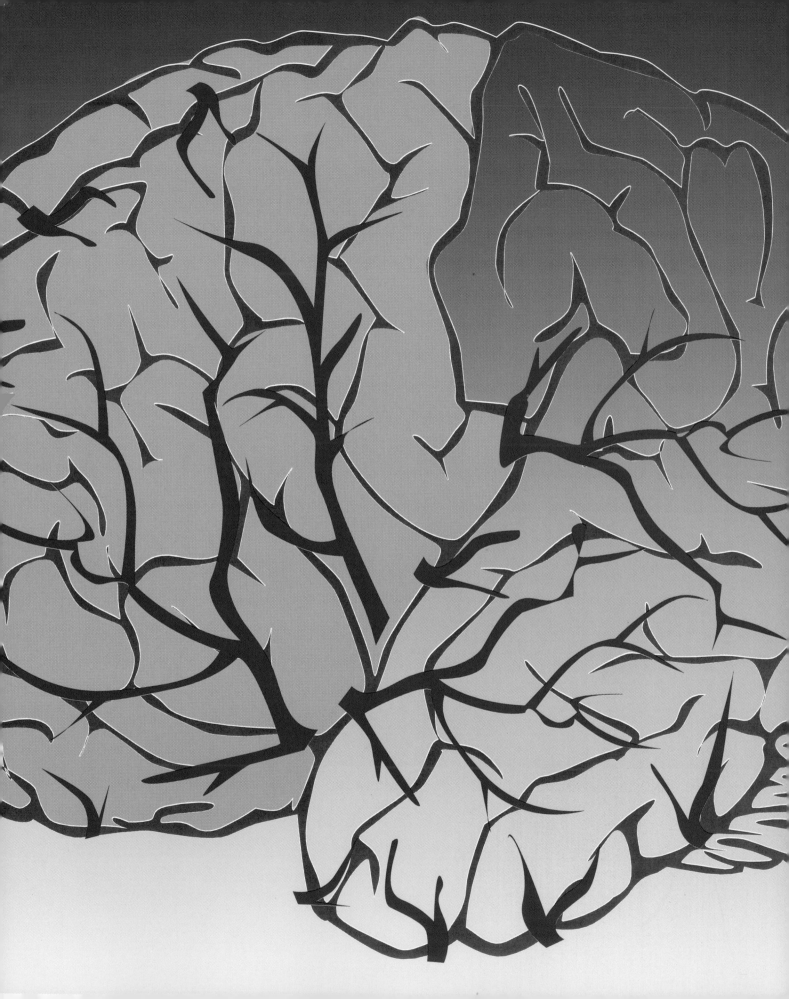

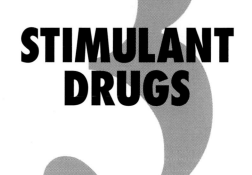

STIMULANT DRUGS

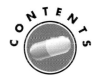

CONTENTS

THE DRUGS DISCUSSED in this section are all central nervous system (CNS) stimulants. To emphasize their common effects, this book groups the stimulant drugs more broadly than is sometimes done. There are at least three drugs among the stimulants that are familiar in some way to just about everyone, namely nicotine, cocaine, and caffeine. All three are natural products, and all three have long been used by humans for their particular stimulant properties. Of these three, only cocaine is a controlled substance. *Controlled substances* are drugs that have been identified as having abuse potential. They are also under legal restraints for use.

There are subgroups within the category of stimulants, for example amphetamines, which are commonly referred to as speed. The drugs within a subgroup may have chemically related structures and usually act by a similar mechanism. For example, although cocaine and amphetamines are unrelated chemically, their effects occur through related neurotransmitters.

Like other drugs of abuse, stimulants activate the brain's reward circuit. Cocaine is outstanding in its specificity for the reward circuit and also in its intensity of effect in the circuit. These factors make the psychological and physical dependence produced by cocaine greater than that for any other drug.

Amphetamines, their derivatives, and related compounds, share several similar effects with cocaine. One difference between the two is that the intensity of effect for the amphetamines may be less, but the duration is always longer. Another difference is that the frequency of certain side effects—psychosis, for example—is higher for amphetamines. Amphetamines also have some completely unique side effects. For example, some of the amphetamines and derivatives are *neurotoxic*—they can cause neuron death.

Some would argue that nicotine has at least as much attraction for use and abuse as cocaine. Whether this is true or not, societal acceptance and legal access have made the number of users impressive. Nicotine is treated like alcohol and its possession and use are legal, but only for adults.

Nicotine clearly produces a response in the reward circuit, placing it in the company of the other drugs that are abused. Nicotine tolerance also occurs, although the increases in smoking to maintain an effect are usually very slow, especially compared with other stimulants such as cocaine or amphetamines. An excessive amount of a behavior that normally activates the reward circuit, such as overeating, is sometimes used in place of nicotine. This may contribute to the weight gain that is often a problem for those who do manage to quit. Cocaine has a much more intense impact on the reward circuit than does nicotine. For this reason, substituting behavior that is not related to drug activity is not effective.

Of the stimulants discussed in this section, caffeine has the widest use. Its effects are clear and well-known, but more subtle than those of the other stimulants. Caffeine has been openly accessible and usable by all, including children. Indeed, caffeine is a common additive to soft drinks. Some schools have prohibited the use of caffeine during school hours due to concerns that caffeine abuse may become a problem.

The current concerns about adverse health effects associated with caffeine consumption are based on small increases in blood cholesterol, an associated risk of cardiovascular disease, and a risk of reproductive abnormalities. In survey data or lab studies, these occur at caffeine levels well above those for average intake. Average intake in the United States is 300 milligrams (about one-hundredth of an ounce) or less daily. This is an amount found in about 2–3 (average strength) cups of coffee, 6–8 cups of tea, 5–10 twelve-ounce colas or 9–10 cups of hot chocolate. The level of caffeine consumption is similar in Western Europe, but averages about 50 milligrams daily in other parts of the world. Moderation may be the key to controlling the adverse effects associated with this drug.

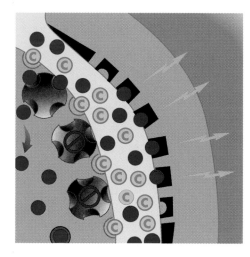

CHAPTER 10

How Cocaine Works

COCAINE IS PRESENT in all parts of the South American shrub *Erythroxylon coca*. Chewing coca leaves with an acid source such as lime juice makes cocaine available for absorption. Coca chewing was already in practice among Andean Indians for at least 5,000 years at the time Spanish explorers arrived in the sixteenth century. Coca is still chewed legally in Latin America, mainly in the Andes. No significant abuse problem occurred for a long time due to low cocaine content in the leaves and low absorption of the total amount that was available. Cocaine extraction in 1860 made high doses possible, particularly by inhalation (snorting) and intravenous injection. (The form in which cocaine is usually purified is not suitable for smoking.)

Cocaine use increased significantly by the 1880s. By the 1890s reports of abuse were frequent. Cocaine use was initially viewed as safe and it was considered a potential panacea. For example, Sigmund Freud (1856–1939), an intravenous cocaine user, recruited his friend and fellow physician, Carl Koller, into personal explorations of cocaine's effects in an unsuccessful attempt to cure another friend's morphine dependence. Cures for morphine and alcohol abuse were common claims for cocaine-containing patent medicines. Koller recognized the local anesthetic action of cocaine and implemented its use in eye surgery.

Coca-Cola began as one of many cola-flavored beverages, also touted as a tonic. In 1906, the company switched to coca leaves from which the active ingredient had been removed. Coca-Cola's decision heralded legislation that forced cocaine's removal from other merchants' products. Drug laws passed in the early 1900s that applied to coca/cocaine ended coca leaf importation. However, cocaine remains available for legitimate medical uses.

Cocaine can inhibit peripheral neurons that communicate pain signals, causing a numbing, or local anesthetic, effect. Numbing of the tongue during coca chewing provided a clue to this action. Cocaine's high-dose toxicity symptoms may be due to local anesthetic actions in the brain. Cocaine inhibits re-uptake of the neurotransmitters norepinephrine, serotonin, and dopamine. Re-uptake inhibition prolongs and intensifies neurotransmitter effects within and outside the central nervous system (CNS).

Cocaine increases dopamine in the brain's reward circuit, causing intense pleasure and reinforcing drug-taking. Increased alertness and movement, altered thinking, and appetite suppression are also cocaine effects in the CNS that involve additional neurotransmitters. Cocaine-induced appetite suppression can cause profound weight loss, even malnutrition.

Cocaine increases heart rate and force by increasing the amounts of norepinephrine in neural junctions on the heart. Increased norepinephrine is also the mechanism by which cocaine constricts blood vessels, increases blood pressure, and decreases blood flow to organs. The consequences of increased amounts of norepinephrine include heart attacks, strokes, organ failure, and damage to unborn babies. An acute toxicity syndrome that includes psychosis, seizures, elevated temperature and blood pressure, and more can occur with acute or cumulative high doses during a run of use. A run of use is a use pattern in which the drug is taken repetitively until it is used up.

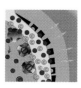

Repeated use causes cellular adaptations that usually result in tolerance but occasionally cause sensitization (an increasing possibility of seizures is an example of sensitization). Tolerance is so rapid that a single use significantly decreases the euphoria of subsequent doses. Withdrawal symptoms are mild and include depression and increased sleep and appetite.

The current cycle of cocaine abuse has reportedly peaked. However, cocaine abuse, alone and with other drugs such as heroin (speedballs), phencyclidine or PCP (spacebase), and alcohol, is still significant. The consequences of cocaine abuse remain extremely serious. These include sudden deaths and toxicity symptoms. Treatment of acute cocaine toxicity is complex and symptomatic; there is currently no specific antagonist as there is for narcotics.

Common street names for cocaine include coke, royalty, girl, lady, snow, gold dust, crack, and rock.

How Cocaine Produces Effects

The effects of cocaine are due to increased levels of the neurotransmitters dopamine, norepinephrine and serotonin. Inhibiting re-uptake of these neurotransmitters intensifies and prolongs their effects within and outside the CNS.

2 Re-uptake occurs by means of special presynaptic carriers. The neurotransmitter binds to a carrier, moves to the inside of the terminal, and is released.

1 Cocaine takes effect when it binds with its receptors. This interaction blocks the function of re-uptake carriers on the axon terminal.

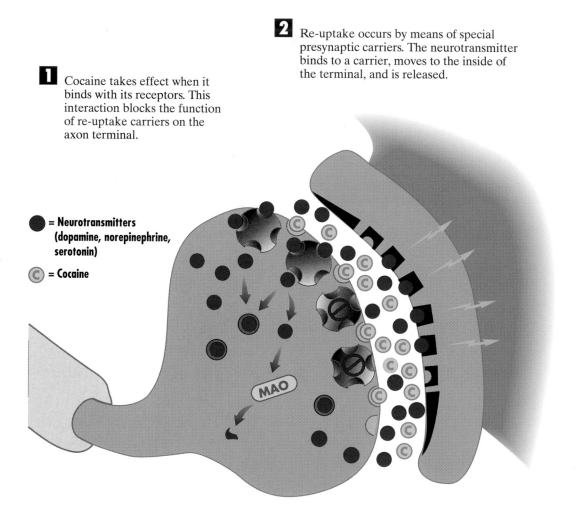

● = Neurotransmitters (dopamine, norepinephrine, serotonin)

ⓒ = Cocaine

3 The activity of dopamine, norepinephrine, or serotonin in a synapse (neuron-to-neuron junction) or a neuro-effector junction (neuron-to-tissue, organ junction) is stopped primarily by re-uptake into the terminal from which it was released. Under most conditions, only very small amounts of these neurotransmitters are removed from the synapse by enzyme degradation.

5 Binding of cocaine to its receptors prevents the re-uptake of neurotransmitters . The amount, duration, and effect of neurotransmitters in synapses and junctions throughout the body increases.

4 Most of the neurotransmitter taken up into the terminal is returned to vesicles (by a second carrier associated with the vesicle) for reuse. While in transit between re-uptake and restoration to a vesicle, a small amount may be broken down by an enzyme (MAO) present in the terminal.

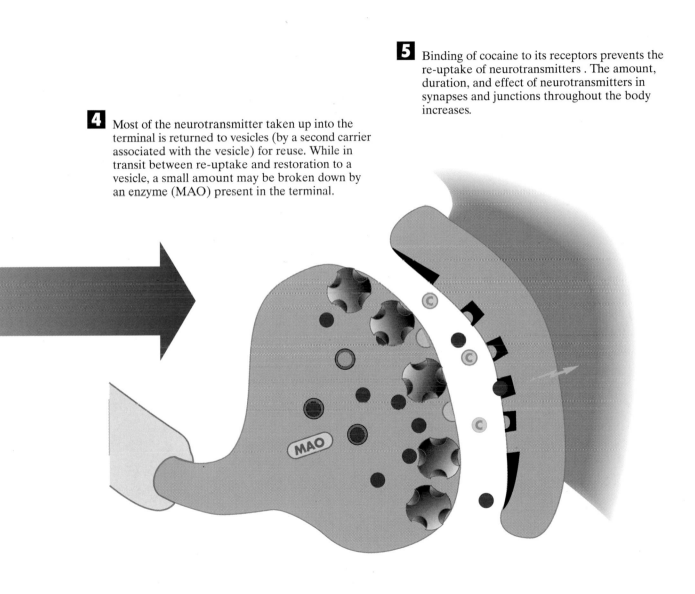

6 Repeated use of cocaine causes short- and long-term cellular changes. Short term, the amount of neurotransmitters in the vesicles decreases. This change can contribute to a rapid type of tolerance known as tachyphylaxis. Slower cellular changes also occur and contribute to longer-term tolerance. For example, the number of neurotransmitter receptors on target cells and cocaine receptors on terminals decreases. Re-uptake carriers, in contrast, increase.

The Acute and Chronic Effects of Cocaine

Cocaine significantly affects the brain, regardless of the form in which it is taken. Its presence in the body increases the activity of dopamine in the reward circuit, causing euphoria and reinforcement of drug use. Increased neurotransmitter activity occurs in other brain areas, including the cortex and limbic and reticular activating systems. Specific neural effects range from altered mood, memory, and pain sensation and awareness, to paranoid psychoses, seizures, and death. The latter effects increase with dose and duration of use.

How cocaine is used influences its effects. The more rapidly the cocaine is absorbed and delivered to the brain, the greater the euphoria experienced will be. Reinforcement and the possibility of side effects are also greater.

Chewing coca leaves releases cocaine slowly and continuously. Coca leaves contain only about 1% of cocaine by weight, so relatively small amounts are swallowed during chewing. Swallowed cocaine is absorbed slowly. These factors contribute to low, steady levels of cocaine in the blood from leaf-chewing, and thus significantly less euphoria, than for cocaine obtained through other commonly used routes.

Time to Brain by Common Abuse Routes

Smoking = 6 – 8 secs.
Intravenous = 10 – 20 secs.
Snorting = 3 – 5 min.

Chewing produces lower, steady level of drug

Cocaine is purified from leaves as a salt (hydrochloride). Cocaine in this form can be absorbed by inhalation and can be used for injection. Inhalation (snorting) produces rapid levels and also rapid decline. Levels in the brain sufficient for effect are reached within 3 to 5 minutes. The effects of intravenous injection are even more rapid, in under a minute.

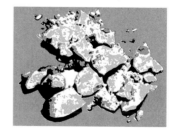

Smoking produces effects in an even shorter time than intravenous use, usually in under 10 seconds. Two forms of cocaine base have been used for smoking, freebase and crack. These forms are chemically identical, but are prepared differently. *Freebase* refers to base isolated in ether after treatment of water-dissolved salt with ammonia. The ether is evaporated to obtain a very pure, solid drug. *Crack* refers to the nonsalt form of cocaine that is isolated in water solution after treatment of water-dissolved salt with baking soda (sodium bicarbonate). The dried chunks have some impurities and also contain bicarbonate. The latter pops or cracks when heated, accounting for the name.

Administration routes affect organ toxicity as well as reinforcement intensity. Smoking cocaine provides rapid, intense effects that can damage the lungs. The user may not even be aware of the damage due to the local anesthetic effect of the smoke. Asthma, bleeding in the lungs, or, worse, fatal lung edema or crack lung may result. Crack lung, a complex of symptoms that includes coughing up blood and fluid accumulation in the air sacs, may represent cocaine hypersensitivity or allergy. Air sacs are frequently ruptured by the smoker's practice of forcibly blowing smoke into another's lungs to increase the effect. Scarring and decreased function are long-term general consequences of smoking cocaine. Other routes also have risks: Injection can lead to infections, including AIDS; inhalation (snorting) can lead to an ulcerated or perforated nasal septum and/or chronic sinusitis.

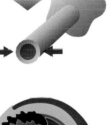

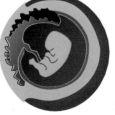

Cocaine crosses the placenta and reaches a developing fetus. Any or all of the effects described above can also occur in the fetus. Growth before birth may be lessened due to constriction of blood vessels in the placenta. The placenta may detach early, one of several factors causing increased premature deliveries. Altered neuron function or neural connections can result from exposure during critical stages of brain development.

A division of the peripheral nervous system (PNS) regulates heart rate and force, the diameter of blood vessels, and even factors that control visual acuity, such as pupil size and lens thickness. One subdivision of the PNS communicates through norepinephrine. Cocaine increases the effects of this subdivision. Cocaine increases constriction (decreases diameter) of blood vessels throughout the body and increases blood pressure. Constriction can occur in some vessels to the point that blood flow is very limited or even stops, a condition known as ischemia. Ischemic tissue does not receive enough oxygen or nutrients and becomes damaged and may even die. Cocaine may also cause *platelets*, small circulating elements of blood, to clump together and/or stick to blood vessel walls. Stimulated platelets release additional constrictors and other chemicals. Platelets can thus cause or worsen ischemia.

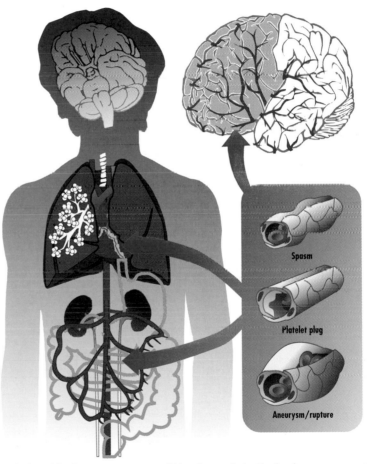

Constriction, blockage, or rupture of blood vessels in the brain can cause strokes or cerebral atrophy, which is a result of progressive death of neurons in the cerebral cortex.

Acutely, cocaine increases heart rate and force. Cocaine can also cause heart attacks through the effects on blood vessels described above. Altered rhythm can occur from increased norepinephrine or from effects of chemicals released from platelets. Fatal heart attacks and dysrhythmias can occur even in the young. Long-term increased blood pressure, decreased blood supply, and increased exertion can lead to a weakening of the heart (cardiomyopathy) similar to that seen in chronic alcoholism.

Cocaine can affect blood vessels in multiple organs. Ischemia, or lack of blood supply to the bowels can cause bowel death and shock. Kidney failure can result from similar effects on blood vessels and/or secondary to destructive effects of cocaine on muscle cells.

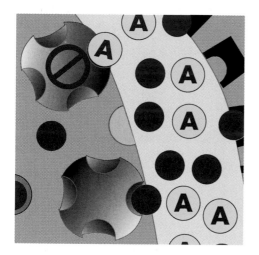

How Speed and Its Relatives Work

THE AMPHETAMINES ARE a group of synthetic chemicals that structurally resemble the neurotransmitters dopamine, serotonin, and norepinephrine. Some of these have primarily stimulant activities and are discussed here; others have a significant component of hallucinogenic activity and are discussed with LSD in Part 4. The first to be synthesized, in 1927, was amphetamine itself. Methamphetamine, or speed, was synthesized next, followed by two closely related compounds given the acronyms MDA and MDMA. All of these have been and continue to be abused.

Amphetamine, also known as an upper or bennie, was first used as a nasal decongestant in Benzedrine Inhalers between 1932 and 1949. Amphetamine was replaced by a compound that does not cause central nervous system (CNS) effects. Amphetamines have also been used for depression; appetite suppression and weight control; sleep substitution to extend performance; narcolepsy (periods of uncontrollable sleep); and childhood hyperactivity (attention deficit disorder). The treatment of narcolepsy and hyperactivity are the only medical uses remaining.

Amphetamine use was widespread among soldiers during World War II. Rampant abuse followed the war in Japan, Sweden, and some other European countries. The U. S. military in Vietnam used amphetamines extensively, but a significant abuse problem in the U. S. began only after physicians started prescribing amphetamines as a treatment for heroin dependence. An abuse explosion occurred in the United States during the 1960s, especially on the West Coast. Abuse remains a significant problem: A large portion of legally produced amphetamines are diverted to illegal use.

Amphetamines are absorbed after ingestion, inhalation (snorting), injection, or smoking. As in the case of cocaine, the more rapidly a dose is delivered, and the higher the level achieved, the greater is the euphoria, or rush. Amphetamine effects are essentially indistinguishable from cocaine effects except by chemical testing. The mechanisms of effect differ somewhat; the durations of action and toxicities differ significantly.

Amphetamines produce long-lasting effects; methamphetamine can be effective for nearly a day. Amphetamines enter axon terminals and displace the associated neurotransmitters, which then leak from the terminal and interact with their receptors. Amphetamines are very fat soluble; they accumulate in the brain and also in fat cells with repeated use. Levels of amphetamines in the brain may exceed by 10 times the levels in the blood. The long duration and accumulation account for a high occurrence of toxic psychoses. Adrenalin causes the effects associated with fear and the fight-or-flight reflex. It also releases amphetamines from fat cells. Release from fat may be the reason for a known increase in drug effects such as paranoid psychosis and physical aggression due to fear or other excitement in chronic users.

Amphetamines, particularly methamphetamine, MDA, and MDMA, are potentially neurotoxic at doses that are only two to three times the minimum dose to produce psychologic effects. Long-term inability to experience pleasure may be due to neuron death. It has been suggested that movement disorders similar to Parkinson's disease may result from amphetamine use because of chemical similarities to another neurotoxin, MPTP. Thus far, a firm connection has not been made.

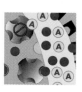

Ephedrine and cathinone, close relatives of the amphetamines, occur naturally. Purified ephedrine has been used as the starting material for synthesis of the nonnatural compounds. Ephedrine is extracted from the shrub *Ephedra sinica*. Ephedra leaves have been used in stimulant teas and traditional medicines such as the Chinese drug Ma Huang for thousands of years. Ephedrine is still used today in a nonprescription preparation for mild asthma. Cathinone occurs in the shrubby tree *Catha edulis*. Dried *Catha edulis* leaves, or khat (qat), have been used as a stimulant and social facilitator in the Middle East in particular for at least a thousand years. Methacathinone, a chemical derivitive of cathinone known by the street name *cat,* has recently increased in use. Like methamphetamine, it is very long acting and thus has increased risk of adverse effects and reactions.

Cellular adaptations occur with the repeated use of amphetamines. These adaptations cause tolerance and account for withdrawal symptoms. Withdrawal symptoms are relatively mild and are similiar to those for cocaine: excessive sleep, increased appetite, and behavioral depression.

How Amphetamines Produce Effects

Amphetamines act on neurons that function with the neurotransmitters dopamine, norepinephrine, and serotonin in both the central nervous system (CNS) and the peripheral nervous system (PNS). The CNS effects are very pronounced because these drugs are very soluble in lipid (fat), and they can enter the brain easily and can even accumulate there. Many CNS effects, particularly in the reward circuit, are due to dopamine. Effects outside the CNS are largely due to norepinephrine.

1 After amphetamines enter axon terminals, they are taken up into the vesicles that store the associated neurotransmitters. This causes the neurotransmitters to be displaced, or leak, from the vesicle into the terminal and from the terminal into the synapse. The displaced neurotransmitter is "extra," and causes an increase in effects.

The action of the particular neurotransmitters released by the amphetamines is ended by re-uptake into the terminals and vesicles. The amphetamines themselves may also inhibit re-uptake.

The enzyme MAO (monoamine oxidase) present in the terminals can break down neurotransmitters outside of storage vesicles. The amphetamines inhibit MAO so that the neurotransmitter remains intact and leaks from the terminal.

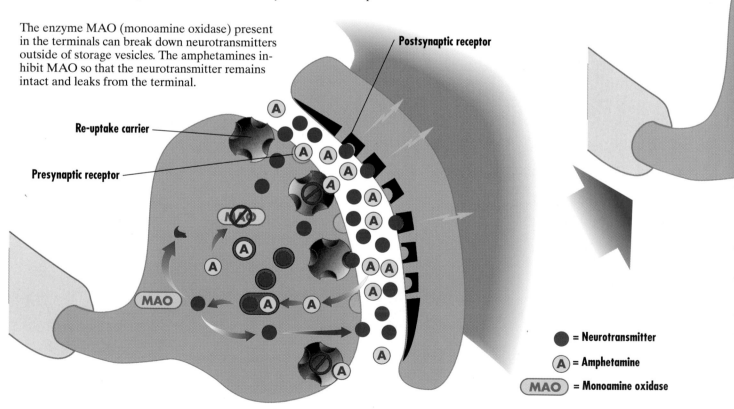

Postsynaptic receptor

Re-uptake carrier

Presynaptic receptor

● = Neurotransmitter

Ⓐ = Amphetamine

(MAO) = Monoamine oxidase

The interaction of neurotransmitters with their receptors serves as a signal to the neuron that no more neurotransmitter should be released. *Blocking* these autoregulatory receptors blocks this signal, causing more neurotransmitter to be released. Amphetamines may block these receptors.

Depleted vesicle

3 Amphetamines may be neurotoxic at doses only two to three times higher than the minimum doses used for euphoria. Even a single dose can cause neurotoxicity, so repeated use, with higher doses resulting from tolerance, presents serious risk. The terminals of damaged neurons swell and break down over time and the neuron itself dies. There appears to be some recovery by regeneration, but whether these new neurons are normal or connect normally to other neurons is uncertain.

2 Repeated use of the amphetamines can deplete neurotransmitter vesicles, which limits their effects. Cellular adaptations also occur, including changes in the number of neurotransmitter receptors and re-uptake carriers.

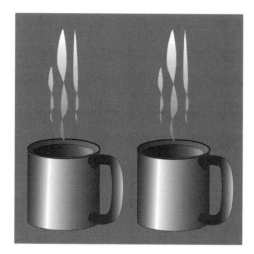

Coffee, Tea, and Cola: How Caffeine Works

CAFFEINE IS THE most widely used and, depending on definitions of abuse, abused legal stimulant in the world. Diverse plants containing caffeine have been used by equally diverse cultures worldwide. Caffeine is most commonly associated with coffee and cola drinks, which contain caffeine extracted along with flavoring from natural sources (coffee beans and kola nuts, respectively). Tea contains significant amounts of caffeine and theophylline, while chocolate (cocoa) contains relatively low amounts of caffeine and theobromine. Theophylline and theobromine are chemical relatives of caffeine; theophylline in particular acts very similarly to proportionate amounts of caffeine.

Coffee beans were probably eaten during the Paleolithic period (c. 2,000,000–10,000 B.C.), long before they were roasted, ground, and extracted with hot water to produce a beverage. The hot drink coffee was first consumed in current Arabic territories around A.D. 1000. Tea beverages originated in China about 2700 B.C. or even earlier. Bitter, unsweetened chocolate drinks were already favored by Montezuma's Aztec nation at the time the Spanish arrived in the 1500s. Similar concoctions were subsequently consumed in Europe, but, thanks to Swiss nuns, were eventually converted to palatable sweet beverages, and related confections in the late 1800s. Modern cola-flavored beverages are likewise introductions of the late 1800s–early 1900s.

Coffee initially was used to facilitate staying awake during long religious events and to allow study during the cool nighttime. Coffee's effects caused some users to abandon khat, another popular stimulant, that is related to the amphetamines.

Caffeine does not produce true euphoria, but it does produce psychologic dependence, increased alertness, and improved motor and mental performance, especially in the fatigued. These effects, along with some of the toxic effects of high doses—for example, agitation and even convulsions—occur mainly by blockade of adenosine receptors. Adenosine is an autoregulatory local hormone that modulates (usually inhibits) the function of most body cells.

Adenosine receptors are usually under some influence of adenosine, and the amount of caffeine in 2 to 3 cups of coffee blocks up to 50% of adenosine receptors. Both of these factors are involved in the potentially bodywide effects of caffeine.

Familiar nonneural effects of caffeine include stimulation of the heart (increased rate and force, and sometimes altered rhythm) and diuresis (increased urine volume). Dilation of airways is a less familiar effect that occurs to an even greater extent for theophylline, which is used in the treatment of asthma. Very high caffeine intake can cause *caffeinism*, a complex of anxiety, irritability, and depression, and a pattern of various hormones in blood usually associated with severe stress.

Cellular adaptations occur with chronic use, causing tolerance to the effects that caffeine produces. A mild withdrawal (lethargy, irritability, headache) can occur with prolonged intake of 600 milligrams (6 cups of coffee) or more daily. Adenosine reportedly increases nicotine's cardiovascular effects. Smokers may be able to offset the increase with high coffee consumption because higher caffeine intake would block more adenosine receptors and limit these effects.

How Caffeine Produces Effects

Neurons store their neurotransmitter in vesicles. A precursor of adenosine, the compound ATP (adenosine triphosphate) is also found in these vesicles and is released along with neurotransmitters. Released ATP is rapidly converted in a series of steps to adenosine, which can then act on any available adenosine receptors.

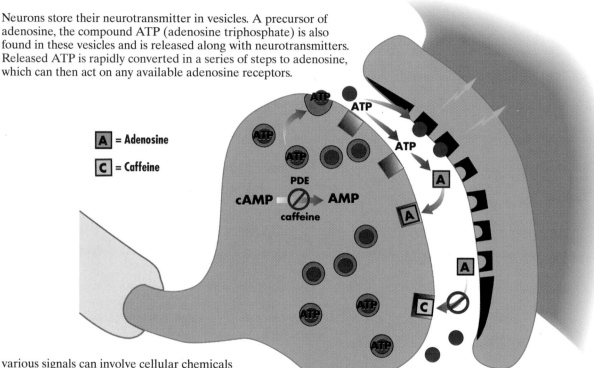

A = Adenosine

C = Caffeine

PDE
cAMP → AMP
caffeine

Cell responses to various signals can involve cellular chemicals known as second messengers. The drug itself—caffeine in this case—can be considered a first messenger. At high levels, caffeine may inhibit the cellular enzyme PDE that breaks down the common second messenger molecule cAMP into another compound, AMP.

Adenosine receptors are located on the axon terminals of neurons. The function of these receptors is feedback regulation of neurotransmitter release. In other words, interaction of adenosine with its receptors is a signal to the neuron that enough neurotransmitters have been released in order to produce an effect. When caffeine blocks adenosine, you feel the effects of the caffeine.

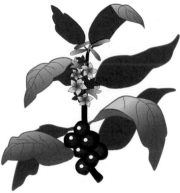

Caffeine produces increased alertness, improved motor and mental performance, especially in the fatigued, and psychologic dependence. These effects, along with some of the toxic effects of high doses such as agitation and convulsions, occur mainly by blockade of adenosine receptors.

Adenosine is a small molecule that functions as an autoregulatory local hormone. Its function is similar to that of a neurotransmitter. Adenosine has effects on or very near the cell that releases it. Most cells contain specific receptors for adenosine. Adenosine interacts with many of its receptors to inhibit some aspect of function of the cell. Caffeine, theophylline, and possibly theobromine, block adenosine receptors and thus limit the effects of adenosine.

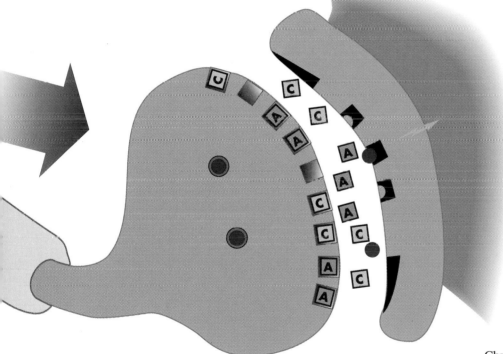

Chronic exposure to caffeine results in cellular adaptations, including increased numbers of adenosine receptors. Tolerance results from these cellular adaptations. Withdrawal effects can occur once tolerance and cellular adaptations have taken place.

Six or more cups of coffee daily constitute chronic, or high, exposure to caffeine.

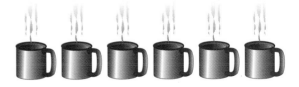

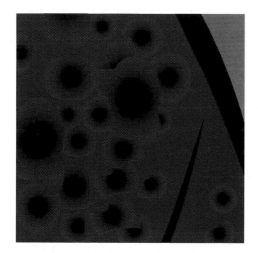

How Nicotine and Tobacco Smoking Work

NICOTINE IS THE main active drug in plants of the species *Nicotiana*. Nicotine is a potent poison that can cause death. Nevertheless, use of nicotine is second only to use of caffeine. Nicotine is considered a gateway drug that may cause some adolescents to abuse alcohol, marijuana, and other drugs. Suprisingly, the Food and Drug Administration (FDA) does not recognize nicotine as a drug, although this may change soon.

Nicotiana tabacum and *Nicotiana rustica* are indigenous to South and North America, respectively. Both were cultivated by native populations, who smoked the leaves in various rituals for many centuries before the arrival of Columbus in North America and the presence of Spanish explorers in Central and South America. Leaf extracts from both plants were also used to kill parasites on and in the body; nicotine is used even today as an insecticide.

N. rustica leaves were brought from North America to Europe in the sixteenth century, introducing both nicotine as a new drug and smoking as a new route of drug administration. Even though *N. rustica* has a higher nicotine content than *N. tabacum*, the qualities of *N. tabacum*, particularly its pleasant taste (relative to other varieties), led to its preferential use and cultivation.

Both *tabacum* and *tobacco* come from the name for a hollow reed used by Native Americans to inhale smoke; *Nicotiana* comes from the name of a French physician, Jean Nicot (1530–1600), who successfully introduced the plant to France. Nicot studied the effects of nicotine extensively and recommended it as a cure-all. From Europe, the practice of smoking tobacco spread rapidly throughout the world.

Pipes were initially the main instruments for tobacco smoking, followed by cigars. Other methods for obtaining nicotine are inhalation of snuff (a fermented, fine tobacco powder) and tobacco chewing. Cigarettes have become popular in the twentieth century, with the increased availability of tobacco and the perfection of mass production devices. Cigarettes have contributed disproportionately to nicotine use and dependence, and to smoking-related disease. Factors such as control of dosing (puffing depth, rate, and so on), availability, affordability, and social acceptance influence the widespread use of cigarettes. The first Surgeon General's Report, issued in 1968, evidenced a correlation between smoking and increased disease and death rates. However, Civil War soldiers were among the first to refer to cigarettes as coffin nails, long before publication of the report.

Nicotine affects all major systems of the body, but is used mainly for its acute stimulant effects on the central nervous system (CNS). Nicotine's desired CNS effects include pleasure, increased alertness, improved mental function and task performance, decreased anxiety, and decreased appetite. Nicotine's additional CNS effects, and some of its non-CNS effects, are due to release of other neurotransmitters and hormones.

The non-CNS effects of nicotine are related to the peripheral nervous system (PNS), which has two main branches. The motor nerves for skeletal muscle are one branch. The other branch consists of two groups of nerves, the sympathetics and parasympathetics, which control automatic systems such as the heart, blood vessels, and various glands. The actions of the sympathetics and parasympathetics are usually opposite. For example, the sympathetics increase, and the parasympathetics decrease, heart rate. Acetylcholine is the neurotransmitter for the motor system. The receptors on muscle are also nAChR. However, nicotine only acts on motor nAChR at toxic concentrations (producing muscle twitches, then paralysis as blockage occurs) unlikely from smoking.

There are two neurons between the spinal cord and an organ, tissue, or gland in both parts of the automatic system. The first neurons synapse on the second within ganglia. Acetylcholine is the neurotransmitter for both neurons in the parasympathetic system and the first neuron in the sympathetic system. However, nAChR receptors occur mainly within ganglia. Nicotine stimulates ganglionic nAChR during smoking; sympathetic effects predominate, increasing heart rate and force, as well as blood vessel tone, which can decrease blood flow to organs as well as increase blood pressure. The hormone vasopressin, released from the CNS by nicotine, constricts blood vessels and increases blood pressure, as well as causes fluid retention due to its effects on the kidney. Nicotine also releases epinephrine (adrenaline) from the adrenal glands, which are really specialized ganglia; epinephrine acts similarly to norepinephrine, increasing heart rate and force, tone of (most) blood vessels, and blood pressure.

Continued exposure results in increased numbers of total nAChR receptors, essentially to compensate for nAChR that are blocked much of the time. Since nicotine releases numerous other neurotransmitters, fewer receptors for these in some brain areas might be expected.

Nicotine acts on specific receptors in the brain's reward circuit. Nicotine increases the amount of the neurotransmitter dopamine in the reward circuit and reinforces its own use, like other drugs of abuse.

Since nicotine is commonly obtained from the smoke of burning dried *Nicotiana tabacum* leaves, other compounds in smoke, such as acetaldehyde, may increase nicotine's effects. Acetaldehyde may increase nicotine use by the use of the same condensation products that occur as a result of alcohol use. Nonsmokers absorb measurable amounts of nicotine and other materials from environmental tobacco smoke and may show negative health effects as a result.

Nicotine is currently used in several (prescription) forms as an aid to stop smoking. Continued smoking-nicotine exposure causes tolerance to early unpleasant effects such as nausea, and also to desired stimulant effects. Tolerance occurs in part by cellular adaptations. Stopping smoking suddenly causes withdrawal symptoms in almost all regular smokers who smoke 15 or more cigarettes per day. Short term, regulated nicotine use may limit irritability, sleepiness, hunger, anxiety, and cigarette craving.

Neoplasms, or cancers, of the lungs (mouth and throat) occur significantly more often in smokers. In fact, certain types of lung cancers occur almost exclusively in smokers. Cancer in other areas is also increased by smoking, including breast, liver/intestines and the prostate. The mechanisms include changes in the structure and function of genetic material, such as formation of DNA adducts by tar derivatives, oxidant damage and more.

Smoking also has adverse affects on females, developing babies, and children. A developing baby receives nutrients and oxygen from its mother's blood as the blood flows through vessels in the uterus. Nutrients and oxygen cross from the uterine blood into the placenta and the baby's blood. Blood flow to the uterus is decreased by smoking, just as it is to other organs. The placenta is damaged in numerous spots by smoking, and is not as attached to the uterus. Babies of smokers are smaller than babies of nonsmokers at all stages of development. Smokers' babies are also more frequently premature than babies of nonsmokers.

Smoking decreases estrogen levels by inhibiting its synthesis and increasing its breakdown. Furthermore, smoking antagonizes estrogen's effects. This causes female smokers to experience menopause earlier and it increases their risk of bone thinning.

Increased allergy symptoms and incidence of respiratory infections and respiratory disease occur in nonsmokers, including children, exposed to environmental tobacco smoke (ETS). Children with a smoking parent also have higher ear-infection rates. ETS has recently been listed as the second highest preventable cause of disease, after smoking itself.

How the Acute Effects of Nicotine Occur

Nicotiana tabacum

Nicotine is very soluble in both water and lipid (fat). It can be absorbed directly and rapidly through the skin in pure form and also from tobacco. Some tobacco products are treated to optimize nicotine absorption from certain locations. For example, chewing tobacco allows for better nicotine absorption from the lining of the mouth than does cigarette tobacco. The liver inactivates swallowed nicotine so that it is only partially absorbed. Tobacco for smoking is treated so that nicotine in smoke is in a chemical form that readily crosses cell membranes in the lung.

Nicotine is the main active drug in plants of the species *Nicotiana*. Nicotine is a potent poison that can cause death. Nevertheless, use of nicotine is second only to use of caffeine. Nicotine is considered a gateway drug that may cause some adolescents to abuse alcohol, marijuana, and other drugs.

During the smoking of one cigarette, and over the course of a day, the receptor blockade increases and the effect of nicotine decreases. Ten minutes is the average amount of time that it takes to smoke a whole cigarette. Each puff from a cigarette produces a nicotine peak, and adds to residual background nicotine. After an initial cycle of increasing use and increasing tolerance, smokers stabilize a use level and pattern that provides nearly continuous effects and no withdrawal symptoms. Smokers maintain their usual nicotine levels by changing the number of puffs and inhalation depth and duration. Therefore, switching to low nicotine cigarettes may not accomplish the goal of reducing nicotine. Desire to smoke starts as nicotine levels drop, and/or in response to behavioral cues (with coffee, after dinner, during times of stress). *Peak seekers* strive for intense effects, evidenced by steep blood nicotine spikes. *Trough maintainers* avoid withdrawal and have a more even, high background blood nicotine. *Long-term chippers* smoke only a few cigarettes per day, have no set blood nicotine pattern and can start and stop at will.

Nicotine in cigarette smoke enters the lungs in association with small particles generated during burning. These small particles contact lung surfaces and nicotine rapidly enters blood and is delivered almost directly to the brain.

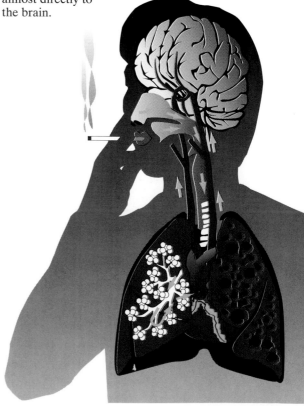

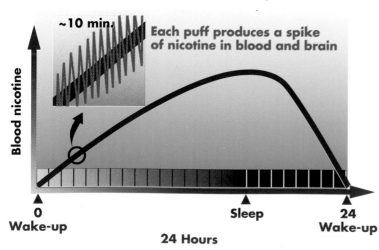

~10 min.

Each puff produces a spike of nicotine in blood and brain

Blood nicotine

0
Wake-up

Sleep

24
Wake-up

24 Hours

1 Nicotine chemically resembles the neurotransmitter acetylcholine. Nicotine acts on specific receptors that are a subset of acetylcholine receptors. The basic effect of nicotine is to increase channels for positively charged chemicals such as calcium. This reaction in turn triggers the release of neurotransmitters. Nicotine stimulates, then blocks its receptors, especially as doses increase.

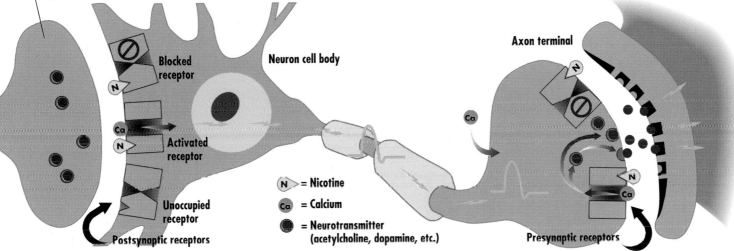

Acetylcholine neuron

Blocked receptor

Neuron cell body

Axon terminal

Activated receptor

N = Nicotine

Ca = Calcium

= Neurotransmitter (acetylcholine, dopamine, etc.)

Unoccupied receptor

Postsynaptic receptors

Presynaptic receptors

2 Nicotine broadly affects the CNS, including the cerebral cortex, through release of neurotransmitters. CNS nicotinic receptors can be postsynaptic or presynaptic. Nicotine action on both types releases neurotransmitters, locally for presynaptic receptors, more distantly for postsynaptic receptors. Released neurotransmitters then act on their own receptors.

3 Nicotine increases the amount of the neurotransmitter norepinephrine in the locus ceruleus by a presynaptic action and dopamine in the reward circuit by a postsynaptic action. Stimulation of the locus ceruleus causes arousal, increases alertness, decreases stress reactions, and improves concentration, all of which may contribute to improved task performance. Increased reward circuit activity causes pleasure and euphoria and, by reinforcing drug taking, contributes to dependency. Reward circuit effects may be amplified by nicotine release of naturally-occurring opiates that originate or are produced within the brain. Nicotine stimulates the brain stem's vomiting center, a problem mainly for beginning smokers.

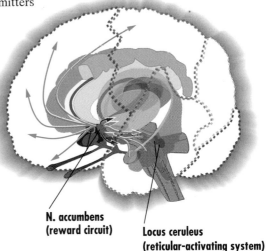

N. accumbens (reward circuit)

Locus ceruleus (reticular-activating system)

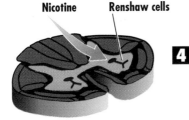

Nicotine

Renshaw cells

4 Nicotine decreases skeletal muscle tone by stimulating spinal-cord Renshaw neurons. Renshaw cells are part of an autoregulatory loop in which motor neurons signal skeletal muscles to contract. Contraction stimulates special sensory nerves in muscle, eliciting neurotransmitter release from their terminals in the cord. This activates Renshaw cells, which in turn release an inhibitory neurotransmitter that decreases motor neuron activity. Muscle tone decrease contributes to the sense of relaxation produced by nicotine.

Chronic Effects of Nicotine and Smoking

The effects of long-term smoking result from nicotine itself and from compounds unique to smoke. There are over 4,000 chemicals in smoke; several have significant adverse health effects. An association between smoking tobacco and increased risk of disease is well established. Smoking is the single largest factor in preventable disease in the United States. Smoking cessation restores most risks to nonsmoker levels within a short time.

5 Cigarette smoke contains chemicals with nicotine that locally irritate and damage the airways and lungs. Cells lining the airways have cilia, small whiplike projections, on their surfaces. Cilia "beat" and move mucus and entrapped particles such as dirt and bacteria up into the throat to be swallowed. Scavenger white blood cells also reside in airways and help keep the lungs healthy. Smoking inhibits cilia and scavenger-cell functions. The consequences include smoker's cough, bronchitis, or inflammation of the airways, and more severe infections.

7 Short-term use of prescription nicotine has been shown to significantly increase the probability that a smoker will stop, and will remain a nonsmoker. Two forms of nicotine are used, nicotine chewing gum and nicotine patches. An obvious advantage of both is lack of exposure to smoke. Patches have the particular advantage of highly reliable and even delivery, no unusual taste or nausea, and lack of ability by the smoker to manipulate nicotine delivery. The gum has the particular advantage that the smoker can manipulate nicotine delivery. Disadvantages include taste and possible nausea from local effects of swallowed nicotine. Other drugs that may be used in the future management of nicotine dependence include specific nicotine and serotonin antagonists.

A layer in the patch controls the rate of delivery and gives the proper dosage of nicotine. Nicotine enters the bloodstream once it has penetrated the surface of the skin.

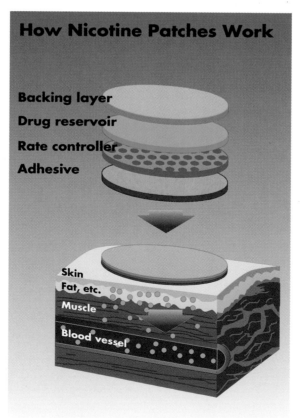

How Nicotine Patches Work

Backing layer
Drug reservoir
Rate controller
Adhesive

Skin
Fat, etc.
Muscle
Blood vessel

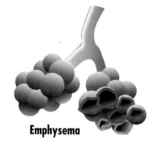

Emphysema

6 Smoking increases chronic obstructive lung diseases such as asthma and emphysema. Contriction of small airways (bronchioles) causes asthma. Emphysema damages a protein that regulates a lung enzyme, allowing the enzyme to damage air sacs. Air sacs rupture and merge, decreasing lung surface area and oxygen transfer. Scar tissue replaces damaged air sacs, decreasing normal elasticity and further decreasing oxygen transfer.

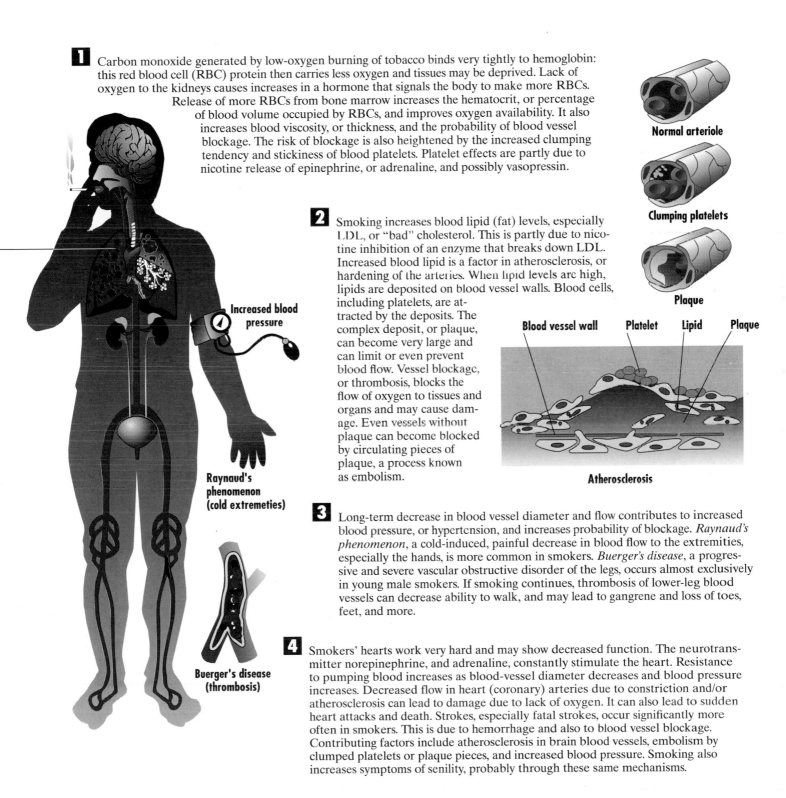

1 Carbon monoxide generated by low-oxygen burning of tobacco binds very tightly to hemoglobin: this red blood cell (RBC) protein then carries less oxygen and tissues may be deprived. Lack of oxygen to the kidneys causes increases in a hormone that signals the body to make more RBCs. Release of more RBCs from bone marrow increases the hematocrit, or percentage of blood volume occupied by RBCs, and improves oxygen availability. It also increases blood viscosity, or thickness, and the probability of blood vessel blockage. The risk of blockage is also heightened by the increased clumping tendency and stickiness of blood platelets. Platelet effects are partly due to nicotine release of epinephrine, or adrenaline, and possibly vasopressin.

Normal arteriole

Clumping platelets

Plaque

Increased blood pressure

2 Smoking increases blood lipid (fat) levels, especially LDL, or "bad" cholesterol. This is partly due to nicotine inhibition of an enzyme that breaks down LDL. Increased blood lipid is a factor in atherosclerosis, or hardening of the arteries. When lipid levels are high, lipids are deposited on blood vessel walls. Blood cells, including platelets, are attracted by the deposits. The complex deposit, or plaque, can become very large and can limit or even prevent blood flow. Vessel blockage, or thrombosis, blocks the flow of oxygen to tissues and organs and may cause damage. Even vessels without plaque can become blocked by circulating pieces of plaque, a process known as embolism.

Blood vessel wall   **Platelet**   **Lipid**   **Plaque**

Atherosclerosis

Raynaud's phenomenon (cold extremeties)

3 Long-term decrease in blood vessel diameter and flow contributes to increased blood pressure, or hypertension, and increases probability of blockage. *Raynaud's phenomenon*, a cold-induced, painful decrease in blood flow to the extremities, especially the hands, is more common in smokers. *Buerger's disease*, a progressive and severe vascular obstructive disorder of the legs, occurs almost exclusively in young male smokers. If smoking continues, thrombosis of lower-leg blood vessels can decrease ability to walk, and may lead to gangrene and loss of toes, feet, and more.

Buerger's disease (thrombosis)

4 Smokers' hearts work very hard and may show decreased function. The neurotransmitter norepinephrine, and adrenaline, constantly stimulate the heart. Resistance to pumping blood increases as blood-vessel diameter decreases and blood pressure increases. Decreased flow in heart (coronary) arteries due to constriction and/or atherosclerosis can lead to damage due to lack of oxygen. It can also lead to sudden heart attacks and death. Strokes, especially fatal strokes, occur significantly more often in smokers. This is due to hemorrhage and also to blood vessel blockage. Contributing factors include atherosclerosis in brain blood vessels, embolism by clumped platelets or plaque pieces, and increased blood pressure. Smoking also increases symptoms of senility, probably through these same mechanisms.

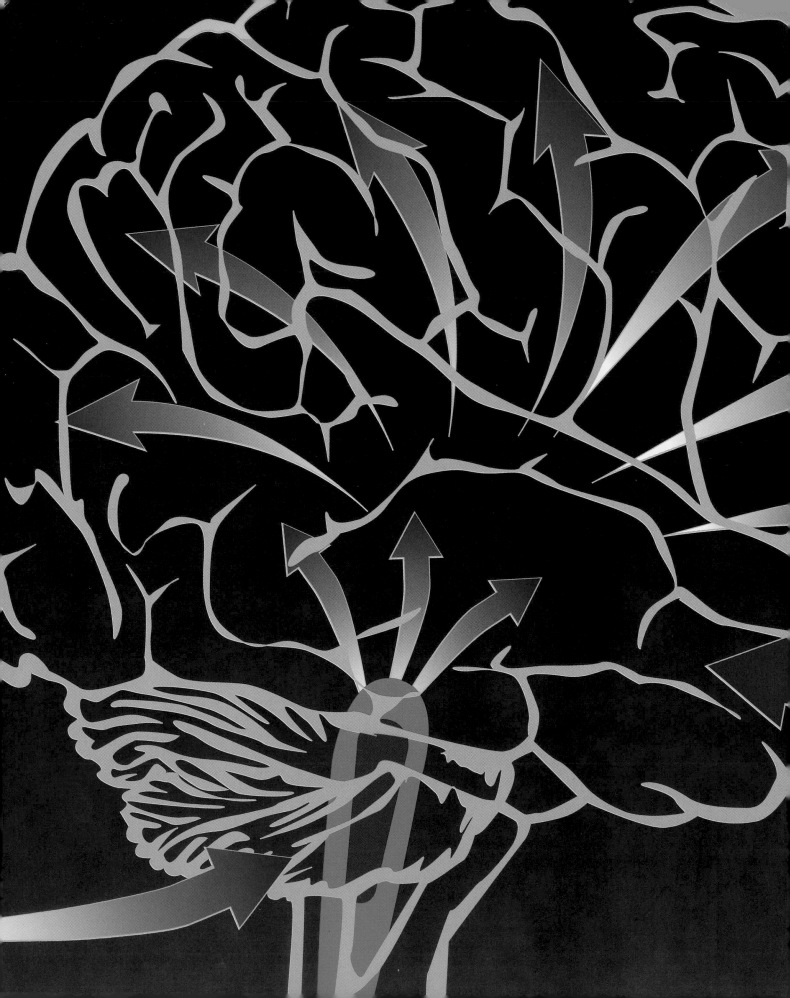

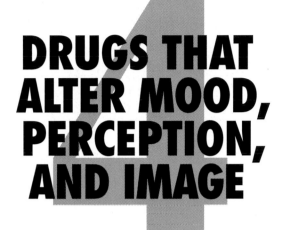

DRUGS THAT ALTER MOOD, PERCEPTION, AND IMAGE

CONTENTS

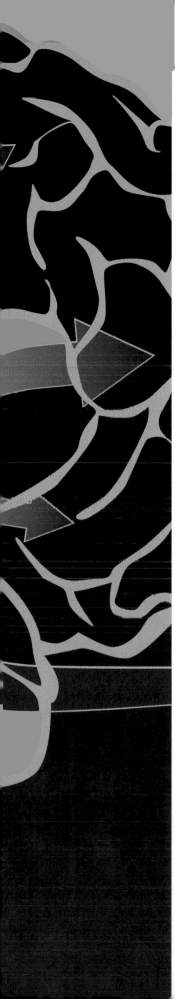

THE ALTERATION OF perception is the common action of drugs discussed in this section. The group name for these drugs has varied in this century. They were known as phantasticants before the term hallucinogens was applied to them. The interest in "mind expansion" that characterized the 1960s made popular the group name *psychedelics* (*psyche* for the soul and *delos* for visible or evident), which was proposed in 1957.

Similarities between the naturally-occurring behavioral disorder of psychosis and the state temporarily induced by these hallucinogens was reflected in other names for this group of drugs: They are also known as psychotogens and psychotomimetics. Recognition of these similarities is critical to understanding and treating mental disease, because of the shared chemical basis of manifested behavior. This discovery has aided pharmacologists in providing some effective and increasingly specific "magic bullets" for psychosis, mania, depression, and other disorders previously ascribed to evil demons or punishment from the gods.

There is a progression from slight modifications of perception to overt hallucinations for all of the drugs in this group. The overall effect depends on the amount of drug that is taken. For some of the drugs, such as marijuana, the progression is slow. Users would experience hallucinations only at very high and uncommon doses. For other drugs, the progression is very rapid, and hallucinations are almost the only endpoint. LSD, partly because of its potency, is an example.

Drugs such as marijuana and the mushroom known as fly agaric have been in use for thousands of years. These and similar drugs have been used in religious and healing rituals, or to arrive at an understanding of the cause, and thus the cure, for physical or psychologic disease. They have also been used to provide escape, pleasure, and power. In fact, the study of some of these older drugs has resulted in new ones that are being used today in much the same manner. For example, analysis of ololiuqui, a drug preparation made from morning glory seeds, led to the synthesis of LSD. LSD has been used for "mind expansion" in much the same way that ololiuqui has been used for hundreds of years in South America.

For most of the drugs in this section, the perceptions being altered concern the outside world. Sensory information—such as color, shape, rhythm, scent, and so forth—from the user's environment is modified during its transit through different areas of the brain under the drug's influence. The final image or sensation produced in the user's mind is therefore different without change in the physical environment. Most often, the perceptual modifications make the final sensory experience more interesting or more pleasant, and thus accomplish the user's goal. Occasionally, however, the drug-induced experience is unpleasant; this is a risk most users are willing to take.

The anabolic steroids fall outside of the caterogy of drugs that were just discussed. Anabolic steroids alter the perception of self-image; the source of altered perception is internal, in the user's mind. There are tangible changes in the user's body that contribute to altered self-image. Other physical and behavioral changes can and do occur, and are accepted risks.

There is general agreement that the perception-modifying drugs are drugs of abuse. Only one drug in this section, PCP, which clearly reinforces its own administration, results in dependence and has a well-defined withdrawal syndrome. Marijuana has some defined, but weaker associations. The drug-seeking behavior for most of the others is almost intellectual, not the driven behavior associated with the narcotics or cocaine.

The pattern of use of many of the perception-altering drugs is unique. Use is occasional, with relatively long intervals between uses; marijuana and PCP are exceptions. Tolerance is so rapid and complete for LSD, for example, that a single dose makes a repeat dose within a day ineffective. For LSD, or any drug causing very rapid and extensive tolerance, direct reinforcement can only occur with use at controlled intervals.

Another consequence of long intervals between doses is that cellular adaptations to the continued presence of drug are not evoked. This is significant because cellular adaptations are an important basis for physical withdrawal effects, and avoidance of withdrawal can reinforce drug use.

Many of the drugs that resemble the neurotransmitter serotonin and the drug LSD (including mescaline, psilocybin, and some of the designer amphetamines) demonstrate cross tolerance. This means that tolerance to one drug leads to tolerance to the other drugs. Therefore, there is no real benefit to switching or rotating use among the drugs.

There is still much to be learned about the mechanisms by which the perception-altering drugs cause their effects. More importantly, there are many remaining questions surrounding the basic chemistry of perception and mood that still need answers.

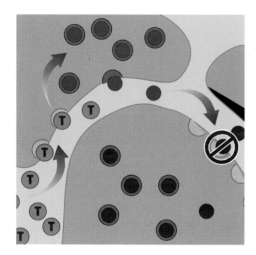

How Marijuana Works

MARIJUANA IS A preparation of dried, shredded leaves from the Indian hemp plant *Cannabis sativa*. Marijuana and other preparations from the plant are sometimes simply called *Cannabis*. Because it resembles lawn clippings, marijuana is also commonly called grass. Other common street names for marijuana include, pot, reefer, weed, ganja, endo, and bud. Hops is also in the hemp family and it has a mild sedative effect, not unlike the effects of small amounts of *Cannabis*. Hops has been used primarily as a flavoring for beer.

Ganja, sinsemilla, hashish, hash oil, and Thai stick are all specific preparations made from the *Cannibis sativa* plant. Ganja and sinsemilla come from the flowering tops of *Cannabis*. Hashish is a brown-black resin obtained by scraping or boiling, while hash oil is a colorless-to-black extract. Thai stick is a compressed product that was favored by the U.S. military during the Vietnam conflict. The various preparations differ in content of the active ingredient, tetrahydrocannabinol (THC) and, to some extent, in how they are used. Marijuana has only 1% to 2% THC, ganja or sinsemilla about 6% to 7%, hashish about 5% to 12%, and hash oil has 20% to 50%. Pure THC is also available in capsule form. Most forms of *Cannabis* are smoked, which adds smoke effects to the drug effects.

Cannabis has been used by humans for perhaps as long as 12,000 years. The first certain written reference to *Cannabis* is in a Chinese document from about 3000 B.C. From China, *Cannabis* spread to India; it is mentioned in Indian writings from about 2000 B.C. The Biblical drug pannag is thought to be *Cannabis*. Pannag is also the source, evolving through the Arabic term *kunnab*, of the Greek name *Cannabis*.

Spanish explorers introduced *Cannabis* as a fiber source to the West in the mid 1500s; it was initially used in making rope. American colonists also grew hemp for fiber from the early 1600s. Medical uses, for pain management, asthma, convulsive disorders, even hysteria, predominated from the 1850s to the early 1900s. Recreational use of marijuana started in Mexico about 1880 when Mexican immigrants, and U.S. soldiers who fought in the Canal Zone or against Pancho Villa, brought it to the U.S. Misstatements about its effects and a purported association with crime resulted in control laws in the United States by the 1930s.

THC produces so many effects that it is difficult to adequately classify it as other than a unique psychoactive drug, affecting the mind and behavior. THC effects occur through specific THC receptors. Low-level effects are similar to those of alcohol—mild central nervous system (CNS) inhibition. When both drugs are taken concurrently, THC effects add to alcohol effects. However, there is no cross tolerance: An alcohol-tolerant individual is fully sensitive to marijuana and vice versa.

Increasing doses produce euphoria by a mechanism that may also involve morphinelike compounds. High doses cause hallucinations and heightened sensory perceptions, especially for vision and sound. The latter resemble the effects of LSD, but there is no cross tolerance between LSD and THC. Decreased coordination, inability to perform multistep tasks, and interference with short-term memory are other common THC effects. Disorientation, paranoid delusions, and panic are rare toxic effects, along with reactivation of schizophrenia and flashback precipitation in previous users of LSD. THC does not produce anesthesia, coma, or death, even at extremely high doses.

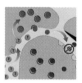

THC reduces pain, nausea, and intraocular (inner eye) pressure. It also has the beneficial effect of relaxing bronchial airways. THC has been approved as an antinausea drug for chemotherapy patients and as an appetite stimulant for AIDS patients. It can also be prescribed for glaucoma (elevated pressure in the eye). Trials for additional clinical uses, in seizure disorders and Huntington's chorea, are in progress.

Decreased testosterone levels, and decreased sperm count and motility, can occur with long-term use. Whether fertility is significantly or permanently affected is unknown. The menstrual cycle is likewise disrupted in females, but again, the long-term significance is unclear.

THC crosses the placenta readily. Dose-related decreases in birth weight and head circumference of exposed newborns have been noted, but no clearly related birth defects have been seen. Babies exposed regularly to THC before birth may show signs of CNS excitation in the neonatal period, including tremors, frequent startle reactions, increased hand-to-mouth activity, and hyperactive reflexes. The long-term persistence of any of these effects is unknown.

Dry mouth and increased heart rate are common side effects of THC. The ability of THC to block some receptors for acetylcholine may account for these effects. Small amounts of acetylcholine are continuously released from the terminals of one branch of the peripheral nervous system. Saliva production is increased, and heart rate is decreased by acetylcholine action on specific receptors at those locations. Blocking those effects would reduce saliva production and increase heart rate.

Tolerance and dependence occur only with very high doses given at close intervals over extended time. Mild withdrawal symptoms occur, including irritability, restlessness, chills, nausea, and possibly vomiting. Amotivational syndrome, characterized by disinterest, poor school or work performance, and memory dysfunction, is a concern with long term, regular use. Recent data indicates significant physical damage to neurons in the hippocampus, a brain area essential to normal memory processes, in long-term, heavy users.

Marijuana is the most frequently used illicit drug in the United States. It is considered a common gateway, or introductory, drug for use of additional drugs.

How THC Produces Effects

1 THC can be absorbed after oral ingestion and through the lungs from inhaled smoke. The composition of *Cannabis* smoke differs from tobacco smoke in ways other than absence of nicotine and presence of THC. *Cannabis* smoke has a very high content of carbon monoxide, tars, irritants, and potential carcinogens. It has been estimated that smoking only a few marijuana cigarettes may cause as much damage as smoking an entire pack of tobacco cigarettes. Another compound in marijuana smoke of particular interest for abuse potential is acetaldehyde, which can chemically react with neurotransmitters to produce condensation products. Condensation products have been implicated in the production of alcohol dependence. Acetaldehyde occurs in tobacco smoke and also appears to increase the dependence potential of nicotine. The acetaldehyde content of marijuana smoke is about 1.5 times higher than in tobacco smoke.

Basal nuclei

Hippocampus

Cerebellum

2 THC receptors in the CNS are numerous, especially in the cerebellum, basal nuclei, and hippocampus, paralleling effects on balance and movement and also memory. The discovery of THC receptors caused a search for a naturally occurring compound that normally acts on them. Very recently the compound anandamide has been identified and shown to interact with the receptors. It is likely that there are additional naturally occurring compounds that can act on THC receptors, and a resemblance to a neurotransmitter may yet be revealed. Additional types of receptors for individual THC effects may also be identified.

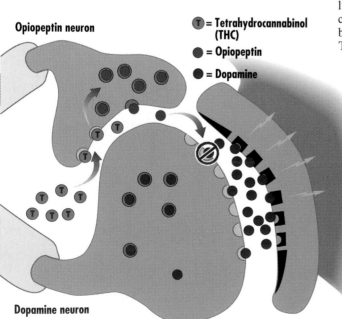

Opiopeptin neuron

- **T** = Tetrahydrocannabinol (THC)
- ● = Opiopeptin
- ● = Dopamine

Dopamine neuron

3 Production of euphoria by THC appears to involve naturally occurring opiopeptins, or morphinelike compounds. THC acts on its receptors, located on an opiopeptin neuron, causing opiopeptin release. The opiopeptin then acts on its receptors on the dopamine neuron in the reward circuit to inhibit dopamine uptake and to enhance the dopamine effect. Evidence supporting this scheme includes prevention of THC euphoria by narcotic antagonists as well as some relief of narcotic withdrawal symptoms by administration of THC.

4 Optimal delivery of THC requires not only inhalation of smoke, but holding the smoke in the lungs for an extended period. The holding process is referred to as pacing. Learning optimal pacing is one reason why the effects of marijuana may be obtained with lower apparent amounts of drug over time. Another reason for apparent increased sensitivity may be accumulation of lipid-soluble THC in the brain and in fat. Repeated daily use can therefore result in very significant accumulation.

5 Continued, repeated marijuana smoking can cause chronic sinusitis, pharyngitis (throat inflammation), and constriction of the airways. The latter can occur even though *nonsmoked* THC can relax airways and has been used for asthma.

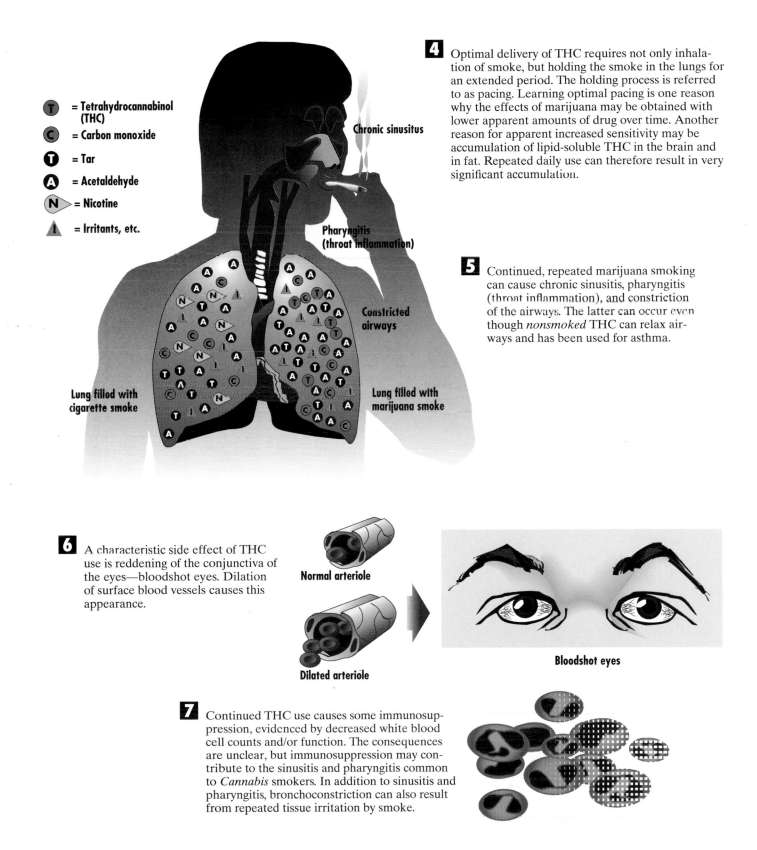

T = Tetrahydrocannabinol (THC)
C = Carbon monoxide
T = Tar
A = Acetaldehyde
N = Nicotine
! = Irritants, etc.

Chronic sinusitus

Pharyngitis (throat inflammation)

Constricted airways

Lung filled with cigarette smoke

Lung filled with marijuana smoke

6 A characteristic side effect of THC use is reddening of the conjunctiva of the eyes—bloodshot eyes. Dilation of surface blood vessels causes this appearance.

Normal arteriole

Dilated arteriole

Bloodshot eyes

7 Continued THC use causes some immunosuppression, evidenced by decreased white blood cell counts and/or function. The consequences are unclear, but immunosuppression may contribute to the sinusitis and pharyngitis common to *Cannabis* smokers. In addition to sinusitis and pharyngitis, bronchoconstriction can also result from repeated tissue irritation by smoke.

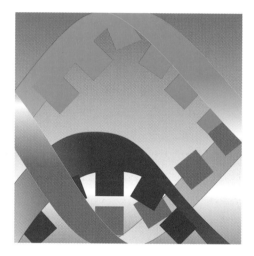

Mushroom Magic: How Mushrooms Work

MUSHROOMS HAVE BEEN used as hallucinogens for thousands of years. Hallucinogenic mushrooms occur within one large family, the *Agaricaceae*, found worldwide. Within *Agaricaceae*, hallucinogenic members are found mainly in the genuses *Amanita* and *Psilocybe*. *Amanitas* include edible, hallucinogenic, and poisonous mushrooms (also called toadstools). Historically, *Amanita muscaria* was used as a hallucinogen mainly in the eastern hemisphere, particularly in the extreme north. However, the Algonquin Indians of North America may also have used *A. muscaria* in rituals. *A. muscaria* is still used in areas of Siberia, and in the West Coast and Northwestern United States.

Amanita muscaria, also known as fly agaric because its juice stuns flies attracted to it, is familiar to most people as the decorative mushroom on cookie jars, kitchen towels, and similar items. It has a red umbrella-shaped cap with white spots and a white stem with a cuplike base.

The drug *Soma*, brought to India thousands of years ago by Aryan invaders, was recently identified as *A. muscaria* by analysis of descriptions in historical records (the Vedic songs). Ancient Vikings used *A. muscaria* to prepare for battle; drug effects were at least partly responsible for their reputation as fearless warriors. Early Greek athletes also fortified themselves for the Olympic games with hallucinogenic mushrooms.

Two closely related hallucinogens, muscimol and ibotenic acid, occur in *A. muscaria*; both stimulate receptors for the neurotransmitter GABA in the central nervous system (CNS). The early effects of *Amanita* are disorientation, incoordination, and sleep, while later effects include intense euphoria, time distortions, vivid visual hallucinations, and mood disturbances that can include rage. Toxic effects can also occur with large doses. *A. muscaria* itself is much less toxic than other *Amanitas* that are highly poisonous, even lethal. Unfortunately, the hallucinogenic, edible, and poisonous types are similar enough in appearance that accidental poisonings are not uncommon.

Two types of *Amanita* poisonings can occur: The first, due to a toxin called muscarine, has immediate onset and is rarely lethal; the second, due to the toxins called amatoxins and phallotoxins, occurs after a delay of many hours and frequently results in death. A rapid onset of toxicity is characteristic of the hallucinogenic varieties and some look-alikes. The effects of muscarine can be prevented with the naturally occurring compounds atropine and scopolamine and their derivatives.

A. muscaria contains small amounts of muscarine. Other *Agaricaceae*, including *Amanitas, Clitocytes*, and *Inocybes*, contain substantially more muscarine, and ingestion can result in greater muscarine toxicity. Muscarine stimulates a subset of receptors for the neurotransmitter acetylcholine. These muscarinic receptors occur in the CNS and also in the peripheral nervous system (PNS). Symptoms of muscarine intoxication include the SLUD syndrome, which consists of salivation, lacrimation (shedding tears), urination, and defecation. Other gastrointestinal symptoms (such as cramping, nausea, and vomiting), constricted pupils, and decreased heart rate and blood pressure may also result.

Psilocybes are common in the Southwestern United States, Mexico, and Central America, where they have long been used in native religious and healing rituals. The Aztecs used *Psilocybe mexicana* (and also the mescal cactus) in religious and other rituals. The name they gave it was *teonanacatl*, or food of the gods. *Psilocybes* are found and used recreationally throughout the United States. They are frequently referred to as "shrooms."

Almost all members of the large *Psilocybe* genus contain the related hallucinogens psilocin and psilocybin. Psilocybin is converted to psilocin in the body. Both compounds are chemically similar to the neurotransmitter serotonin and to LSD. The effects of psilocin are essentially indistinguishable from those of LSD, although psilocin is about 100 times less effective than LSD.

The physical effects of *Psilocybe* use include nausea, sleepiness, blurred vision, dilated pupils, and some increase in muscle tone. Mental effects include increased perception of colors, object definition, patterns and shapes, and afterimages that are longer than usual. The overall experience is usually euphoric, but anxiety may occur and images may become frightening in their intensity or unusual content. All effects are usually over in about 3 hours.

Psilocybes (and the related *Paneolus*, which also contain psilocybin and psilocin) can be found all over the world. *Psilocybes* can be very small, requiring ingestion of a dozen or more dried caps for effect.

How Mushroom Chemicals Produce Effects

Amanita muscaria, also known as fly agaric because its juice stuns flies attracted to it, is familiar to most people as the decorative mushroom on cookie jars, kitchen towels, and similar items. It has a red umbrella-shaped cap with white spots and a white stem with a cuplike base.

Amanita muscaria

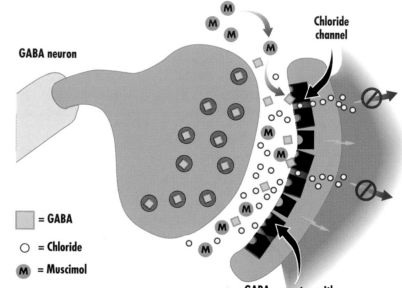

GABA neuron

☐ = GABA

○ = Chloride

Ⓜ = Muscimol

Chloride channel

GABA$_A$ receptor with benzodiazepine binding site; closed chloride channel

The hallucinogenic effects of *A. muscaria* and some less-used *Amanita* are due to (at least) two compounds, muscimol and ibotenic acid. Ibotenic acid is less potent than muscimol, but is converted to muscimol. Muscimol stimulates a subset of CNS GABA receptors, the GABA$_A$ receptors: This increases channels for chloride ions and inhibits neuron function. A GABA$_A$ receptor also has a benzodiazepine binding site, through which the depressant effects of the benzodiazepines (and also alcohol and the inhalants) occur. Almost any neuron may be inhibited by GABA, even without direct GABA innervation. This condition makes muscimol effects more intense than those of other GABA-active drugs, and those effects can also extend throughout the CNS.

The hallucinogenic compounds found in *Psilocybe* mushrooms, psilocybin and psilocin, have chemical structures similar to the neurotransmitter serotonin and also to LSD. These compounds act on CNS serotonin systems and limit serotonin release. When psilocin blocks the release of serotonin, this produces drug effects by decreasing the interaction between serotonin and its postsynaptic receptors. Tolerance to the effects of these hallucinogens occurs rapidly, so rapidly that intermittent use is necessary to maintain effect. Tolerance to psilocybin and psilocin crosses to LSD.

Psilocybe cubensis

S = Serotonin

P = Psilocybin/psilocin

Presynaptic serotonin autoregulatory receptors

Amanita phalloides (or death cap) and *Amanita verna* or *virosa* (or destroying angel) contain two types of toxins: amatoxins and phallotoxins; the phallotoxins are less active in the body. Consumption of even small amounts (less than one half of a death cap, for example) can be lethal in up to 90% of consumers without treatment, and up to 50% even with treatment. Amatoxins cause cell death by interfering with an enzyme, RNA polymerase II, involved in the conversion of the DNA genetic code to cellular proteins. The liver and kidneys are particularly susceptible because of rapid uptake of amatoxins. Rapidly dividing cells, such as the lining of the gastrointestinal system, are also very sensitive. Initial symptoms of intoxication, including severe diarrhea and nausea, occur several to many hours after ingestion, then disappear for several days, only to be followed by symptoms of liver (and/or kidney) failure and possibly death.

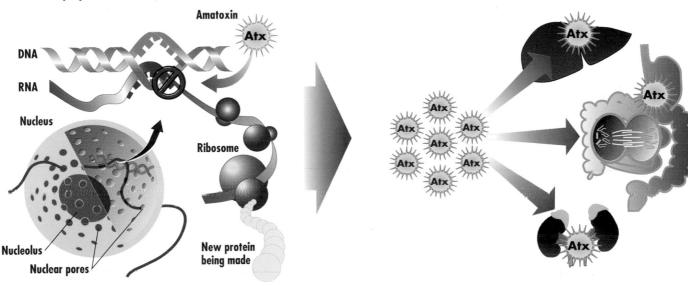

Amatoxin Atx

DNA

RNA

Nucleus

Ribosome

Nucleolus

Nuclear pores

New protein being made

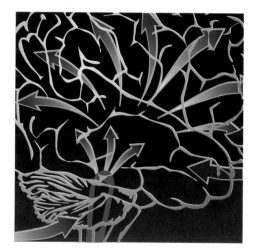

Lucy in the Sky with Diamonds: How LSD Works

LYSERGIC ACID DIETHYLAMIDE, or LSD, is a synthetic hallucinogen with a structure similar to the neurotransmitter serotonin. Although LSD does not occur in nature, other derivatives of lysergic acid are found in nature. For example, lysergic acid amide (LSA) has effects similar to LSD, but is about 10 times less potent. The psychoactive plant preparation ololiuqui, which was studied and led to LSD synthesis, contains LSA.

The fungus *Claviceps purpurea* produces several biologically active derivatives of lysergic acid. These derivatives are collectively called ergot alkaloids. *Claviceps* (also known as ergot), under the right conditions, infects growing rye grain in fields. Grain infection is readily detectable due to characteristic tufts produced in the grain head. During the middle ages and possibly 2,000 years before then, periodic ergot infections of cultivated fields occurred, but the grain was used anyway. Ergotism is the disorder that can result from eating infected grain or its by-products. Ergotism is characterized by necrosis, or cell death, within the extremities.

Some ergot alkaloids are potent vasoconstrictors, which means they narrow the blood vessels. Other ergot alkaloids cause powerful contractions of other smooth muscle—in the uterus, for example. These contractions were sometimes the cause of spontaneous abortions. The ergot alkaloids that cause vasoconstriction or uterine contraction are not psychoactive, but others are, although less so than LSD. Most records of ergotism mention unusual behavioral symptoms, sometimes as severe as overt madness. Ergotism is still occasionally reported.

LSD was synthesized by two Swiss chemists, Drs. Hoffman and Stoll, at Sandoz Pharmaceuticals in 1938. In 1943, Albert Hoffman discovered the effects of LSD firsthand and subsequently reported them. The effects experienced by Hoffman, and others since, are remarkably similar to the symptoms of the well-known psychiatric disorder schizophrenia. An increase in dopamine effect occurs in schizophrenia. Since the symptoms of LSD resemble schizophrenia, increased dopamine may also be involved in this aspect of LSD's effects.

The distinguishing feature between schizophrenia and the effects of LSD is that an LSD user usually knows that the hallucinations are drug-induced, or pseudohallucinations. Recognizing the similarity between drug effect and disease led Hoffman to conclude, correctly, that disorders such as schizophrenia could result from chemical imbalances in the brain. This finding led to the conclusion that solutions to such problems, in the form of specially designed drugs, were possible.

From 1953 to 1966, Sandoz supplied LSD to researchers and clinicians around the world. Distribution was halted, and marketing plans abandoned, when lack of medical application and the potential for abuse were recognized. Timothy Leary, a Harvard faculty member famous for his "tune in, turn on, and drop out" messages during the sixties, was interested in using drugs to achieve "mind expansion." He initiated his studies using the mushroom compound psilocybin, but switched to LSD. His involvement heralded the first public cycle of LSD abuse.

A parallel cycle was occurring simultaneously, but this only came to light after 1975. This nonpublic cycle involved the CIA and the military. The CIA's purpose was to determine the potential utility of LSD in espionage operations. Interest in LSD as a recreational drug has waxed and waned in intervening years; interest has recently increased.

LSD is water soluble, rapidly absorbed after oral administration, and effective in remarkably small quantities. An average dose of 25 micrograms, about one-millionth of an ounce, can produce significant effects lasting 10 to 12 hours. LSD's potency is impressive because brain tissues contain the lowest concentration of LSD of any tissue in the body at all times after the drug is taken.

Another unusual feature of LSD action is its exceptionally rapid induction of tolerance: Doses at close intervals are completely ineffective within about three days. Tolerance to LSD crosses to most other hallucinogens, including hallucinogenic amphetamine derivatives and mescaline; it does not extend to marijuana. Users, therefore, take repeat trips, or doses, at fairly long intervals and do not substitute or simultaneously use other hallucinogens.

The effects of LSD occur in three phases. In the first phase, effects outside the central nervous system (CNS), such as increased heart rate, dilated pupils, and elevated temperature, predominate. These somatic, or body, effects mimic those obtained by stimulation of the sympathetic branch of the peripheral nervous system or the release of adrenalin.

In the second phase, sensory effects predominate, including sensory distortions and pseudohallucinations. The distortions can include persistent visual afterimages, such that previous and current images appear to overlap. A phenomenon known as synesthesia may also occur: Synesthesia refers to a mixing of sensory information so that colors may be "heard" and sounds "seen." The boundaries of the body may also become difficult to distinguish. Despite this, there is usually no major panic in this phase.

In the third, or psychic phase, thought may be disrupted, true hallucinations and even psychotic episodes may occur, and fear of depersonalization and identity loss may become overpowering. LSD has analgesic, or pain-relieving, effects and was at one time recommended for use in terminal cancer patients; despite effective pain reduction, patients refused further doses of the drug after experiencing the effects of the first dose. LSD is also commonly referred to as acid, tab, California sunshine, barrels, contact lens, and white lightning.

How LSD Produces Effects

The cell bodies of serotonin neurons occur in the dorsal and median raphe nuclei of the reticular activating system (RAS) of the brain stem. Projections from these neurons extend to all parts of the brain, including the cerebral cortex and the reward circuit. LSD limits the effects of the neurotransmitter serotonin and can increase dopamine in the brain's reward circuit.

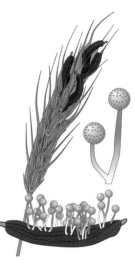

Claviceps purpurea (ergot)

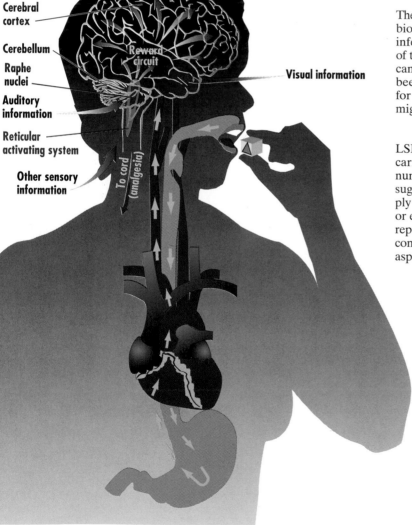

Cerebral cortex

Cerebellum

Raphe nuclei

Auditory information

Reticular activating system

Other sensory information

To cord (analgesia)

Reward circuit

Visual information

The fungus *Claviceps purpurea*, or ergot, produces several biologically active derivatives of lysergic acid. *Claviceps* infects the seed heads of rye and other grains. The tufts of the fungus fall to the ground and germinate. The spores can then infect more grain. Deliberate infections have been done in order to produce chemical starting material for drugs such as ergotamine. Ergotamine is an anti-migraine drug.

LSD is usually sold and taken with the assistance of a carrier. A sugar cube is a common carrier. A calculated number of drops of drug solution are dripped onto the sugar, which is then allowed to dry. The sugar cube is simply placed in the mouth to dissolve and then be swallowed, or even dissolved in a drink. Blotter paper, usually with a repetitive pattern delineating individual doses, is another common carrier. Tablets of nonprescription drugs such as aspirin can also be used as carriers.

Serotonin can interact with both pre- and postsynaptic receptors.

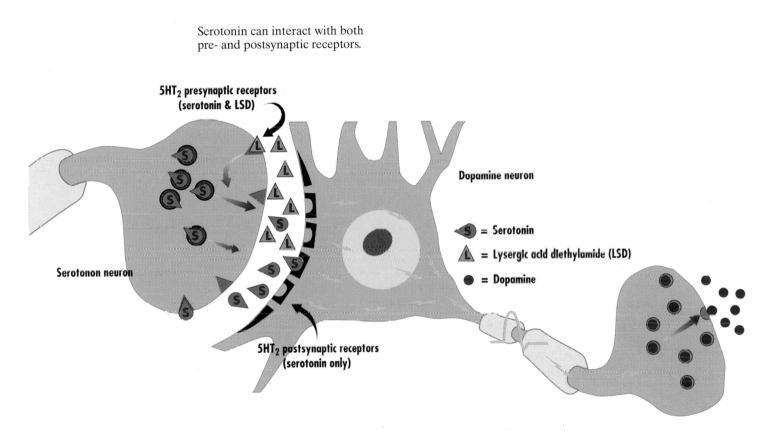

5HT$_2$ presynaptic receptors (serotonin & LSD)

Dopamine neuron

S = Serotonin

L = Lysergic acid diethylamide (LSD)

= Dopamine

Serotonon neuron

5HT$_2$ postsynaptic receptors (serotonin only)

LSD causes many of its effects by activating presynaptic receptors for serotonin in the brain stem, and elsewhere. In the RAS, LSD acts on an autoregulatory subset of serotonin (5HT$_2$) receptors. The effect of stimulating these autoregulatory receptors is to decrease release of serotonin. When this happens, less inhibitory serotonin acts on dopamine neurons in the reward circuit. Subsequently, more dopamine may be released and a sense of euphoria may occur.

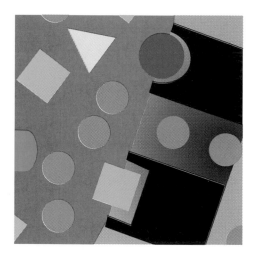

The Fallen Angel: How PCP Works

PHENCYCLIDINE, ALSO KNOWN as PCP and angel dust, was synthesized and developed in the 1950s as a nonbarbiturate, nonnarcotic anesthetic agent. PCP was sold in the San Francisco area as the *PeaCe Pill* (hence PCP) for about a year (1967-68). It appeared in New York about the time it was disappearing on the West Coast, but was known as Hog, signifying its veterinary use. PCP's use, at least as a pure drug, was of as short duration on the East Coast as it had been on the West Coast, presumably because of its many unpleasant side-effects. Although contaminants (occasionally very toxic and even lethal ones) have been a problem, PCP is cheap and relatively easy to synthesize. For these reasons it is frequently combined with, or substituted for, other drugs of abuse. PCP is significantly reinforcing in the reward circuit and has considerable abuse potential.

PCP produces dissociative anesthesia, a sort of semiconscious separation from sensation, without the deep central nervous system (CNS) depression that accompanies other anesthetics. In fact, PCP was of interest because of its potent analgesic (pain-relieving) properties which would also lessen the amount of CNS depression required for anesthesia. No problems were noted during PCP's development, which included numerous tests on various species of animals. Unfortunately, the initial testing led to marketing of an unusable, even dangerous, drug. Parke-Davis patented PCP in the U.S. in 1963. As soon as the drug was used for anesthesia in humans, significant problems occurred, including hallucinations during emergence from anesthesia, delirium, muscle rigidity, and even seizures. The problems were so severe that PCP was withdrawn from legal human use in 1965, just two years after it was patented. However, PCP has remained legally available for veterinary use since 1967, the same year of its first documented illegal use.

PCP can be effective when taken orally. It is also well-absorbed into the bloodstream if snorted or inhaled in smoke. In fact, smoking is a common route of administration for PCP. It can be "dusted" onto burnable substances such as parsley, mint, oregano, marijuana, or even tobacco, which is then rolled into a cigarette or used in a pipe. Mixtures with marijuana, known as Super Grass and Love Boat, are very potent and can produce severe toxic symptoms. A mixture with heroin, known as spacebase, has similar intense and potentially dangerous effects. The usual duration of action of a single average dose of PCP is 4–6 hours. Higher doses can have an effect for a much longer time. PCP is very fat soluble and may accumulate in body fat, and also in the brain, which may increase the duration of action.

Low dose acute and chronic effects of PCP generally resemble those of alcohol, except for a unique, generalized numbness affecting all extremities. Higher doses produce analgesia, sensory disturbances or even sensory block, muscle rigidity, and (perhaps) changes in consciousness or anesthesia. High doses can also cause convulsions, coma, and death.

Perceptual symptoms associated with PCP proceed in stages. They may begin in perceived changes in body image that can include detachment and feeling "out-of-one's-body," followed by visual and/or auditory hallucinations, estrangement, and apathy. Drowsiness, inability to concentrate, and difficulty thinking or verbalizing occur frequently. A sense of emptiness or preoccupation with thoughts of death may occur and acute psychotic episodes are not uncommon. Physical effects, over and above dizziness and incoordination, include elevated blood pressure, rapid pulse, constricted pupils and nystagmus (a rapid side-to-side eye movement), flushing, sweating and drooling, nausea and vomiting, and loss of bladder and bowel control.

Toxic reactions to PCP are not uncommon and include such symptoms as agitation, aggression, violent behavior, and a very unusual blank-stare that can persist even into a coma. A particular problem of an acute toxic reaction is the danger the individual poses to himself as well as others. Accidents such as falls, burns, car crashes, and drowning (in suprisingly small amounts of water) are significant risks, not only because of impaired perception and coordination, but also because of delusional beliefs combined with drug-induced aggression, violence, and lack of sensitivity to pain. Recovery from toxic reactions is usually complete but slow, and the individual may have memory deficits for the time during which recovery took place. The misperceptions, paranoia, aggression, and violence of an acute toxic reaction may last 5 or more days, with characteristic restlessness lasting up to 10 days.

The mechanisms by which PCP produces its myriad effects are still under some debate. Two central nervous system (CNS) receptors account for the majority of PCP's effects. One of these is the sigma (σ) receptor. Other drugs, most notably the narcotics, also act on this receptor. The sigma receptor is involved in dysphoric (unpleasant) drug reactions.

For a long time, sigma receptors were throught to be the primary PCP receptors. However, recent studies have shown that this is not the case. In contrast to the data for sigma receptors, other research has shown that there is a definite correlation between the intensity of PCP effects, particularly the effects that mimic psychosis, and the intensity of its binding to NMDA receptors.

NMDA is an acronym for the name of a compound, N-methyl-D-aspartate, that has been used to study this receptor. The NMDA receptor controls an ion channel and the receptor's function is modulated by several different molecules. Some of these molecules are produced by the cells on which the receptors are found, others from outside the receptor-bearing cell. The NMDA receptor is stimulatory, or excitatory, and is probably involved in neurotoxicity states, such as the severe withdrawal symptoms of alcohol. PCP blocks the NMDA receptor and can even prevent the excitatory neurotoxicity that occurs after certain types of brain injury, for example strokes.

Aspartate and glutamate are the naturally-occurring neurotransmitters that can act on the NMDA receptor; both are classified as excitatory amino acids (EAA). Most neurons in the CNS respond to EAAs. For this reason, removal of (the effects of) EAAs can be compared to stopping all brain activity.

How PCP Causes Its Effects

Two central nervous system (CNS) receptors account for the majority of PCP's effects. One of these is the sigma (σ) receptor, but the most specific receptor for PCP is a complex receptor called NMDA. PCP blocks the NMDA receptor and can even prevent the excitatory neurotoxicity that occurs after certain types of brain injury, for example strokes.

The NMDA receptor is a very widely distributed, complex receptor that has several different binding sites associated with it.

Agents that bind to the NMDA receptor modulate the ion channel that is the functional part of the complex. Binding of two different molecules, an excitory amino acid (EAA) and the amino acid glycine, is required for the channel to be open at times when the membrane potential is also within a certain range. PCP produces its effects when it enters a neuron through an open channel.

Calcium and sodium can also enter the neuron through the open channel. When calcium and sodium are introduced into the cell, this activates, or depolarizes, the cell. This may in turn cause release of additional neurotransmitters, including EAAs, from the cell.

In the open state, magnesium (Mg) can block the channel, as shown. PCP, and related drugs, can also block the open channel by binding to a receptor within the channel. There is some data to show that PCP can even enter cells and bind when the channel is closed, but this is a very slow, and probably not very efficient process.

In addition to interacting with NMDA and sigma receptors, PCP can block re-uptake carriers for the neurotransmitters serotonin, dopamine, and norepinephrine, with somewhat greater effect on serotonin re-uptake. It is unclear whether this effect of PCP reinforces its use, or contributes to dependency.

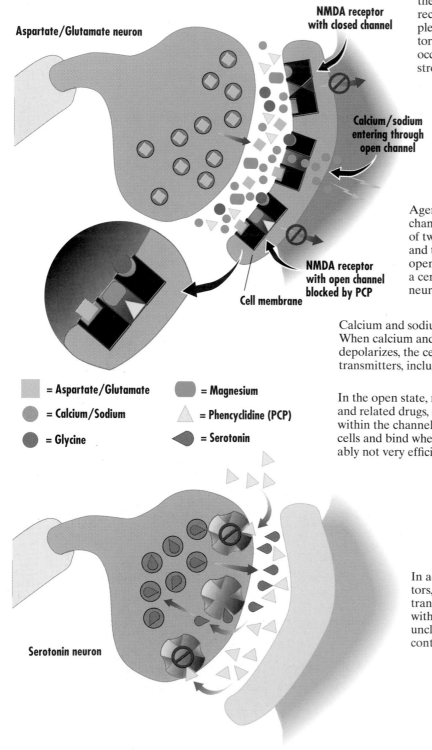

Aspartate/Glutamate neuron

NMDA receptor with closed channel

Calcium/sodium entering through open channel

NMDA receptor with open channel blocked by PCP

Cell membrane

Serotonin neuron

◼ = Aspartate/Glutamate
● = Calcium/Sodium
● = Glycine
⬭ = Magnesium
△ = Phencyclidine (PCP)
⬢ = Serotonin

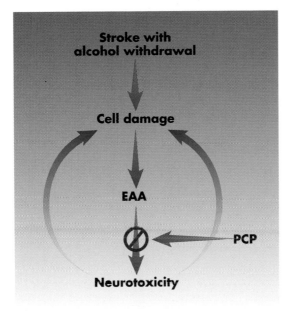

EAAs are thought to be involved in the neurotoxicity, or nerve damage or death, that follows strokes and other injuries. PCP, because it blocks the effect of the EAA, has been shown to prevent post-stroke and post-injury excitation damage. New drugs with PCP-like blocking activity, but lacking PCP's harmful side-effects, are being sought.

High levels of sigma receptors are found in several brain areas, including the cerebral cortex, the cerebellum, and the nucleus accumbens. Binding to these receptors may be one cause of the altered perception and mood that is associated with PCP. This may be due to the role that sigma receptors play in dysphoric and behavioral effects of PCP, narcotics, and other drugs. Curiously, schizophrenics appear to have fewer sigma receptors in the cerebral temporal lobe. This is the location of the limbic system, which is associated with emotion and motivation. This change in the number of sigma receptors may be the result of altered levels of a presently unidentified compound that usually interacts with the receptors.

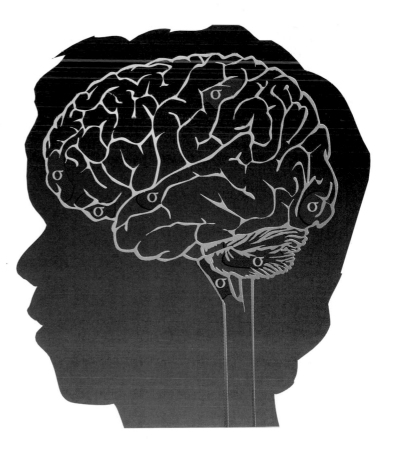

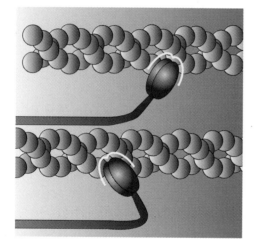

How Steroids Work

STEROIDS ARE NATURALLY-OCCURRING hormones with chemical structures based on cholesterol. There are several types of steroid hormones that are produced at different sites in the body and with differing basic effects. The diverse effects of steroids are essential for normal body functioning. If the body cannot produce steroids, they must be replaced by another source, such as a synthetic relative with similar action, in order to maintain normal function. This is called *replacement therapy*. Some steroids are drugs that are classified as controlled substances.

Hormones are released into blood from specialized gland cells, such as the adrenal glands, which produce the steroid hormones cortisol and aldosterone. The gonads (ovaries and testes) produce the sex steroids estradiol (estrogen), progesterone, and testosterone. There is some cross-over in effects among the steroids. For example, the main function of aldosterone is regulation of salt balance, but cortisol also causes some aldosterone-like salt retention. Also, cortisol and the sex hormones all affect metabolism, although the main effects of the sex hormones are support of gender characteristics and reproductive functions. However, steroids differ in their effects on metabolism. Cortisol is *catabolic*; that is, it favors the breakdown of cellular energy stores and even protein, to provide glucose—effects that can be useful during stress. (By contrast, testosterone is *anabolic*; that is, it favors the synthesis and accumulation of protein by muscle cells, which is the effect of interest for those who misuse steroids.)

By favoring catabolism, cortisol helps keep blood glucose (sugar) available: glucose is a universal energy source that can be used by all cells and is the only form used by the brain in most circumstances. Cortisol levels increase during stress, including the stress of repetitive prolonged exercise. Sustained increases can be detrimental, causing suppression of the immune system, changes in metabolism that resemble diabetes, and loss of muscle mass. Cortisol and naturally occurring anabolic steroids may compete for receptors. This competition may explain in part any beneficial effects of anabolic steroids on muscle performance because it prevents cortisol effects on muscle protein.

The existence of male steroid hormones (androgens) was documented during the late 1800s in simple but elegant experiments. These experiments showed that normal rooster combs and wattles (the structure beneath the beak) can be maintained on castrated roosters by transplanting a testis or giving extracts of testes or male urine, both of which supply tetosterone. By the 1930s, cholesterol and several steroids, including testosterone, had been isolated, and the methods for synthesis of the native product and derivatives had been established. Over 40 synthetic steroids are currently marketed worldwide (many from illegal or veterinary sources). Some are effective orally, others only after injection.

Testosterone has many effects, some even before birth. At puberty, testosterone facilitates growth of bones, muscle, and the vocal cords, which causes characteristic voice deepening. Other effects include beard growth and, eventually in some, baldness. Reproductive structures grow, and fertility and sex drive are established under testosterone's influence. Bone lengthening is also stopped by testosterone: use of steroids before full bone length/height has been accomplished can literally stunt growth.

After puberty, testosterone maintains reproductive structures and functions: A deficiency can cause infertility, disinterest in sex, atrophy of the testes and penis, and so forth. Abuse of anabolic steroids can cause many of these same effects. These deficiency effects are made worse by additive effects of estrogen: Intermediates usually converted to testosterone can be converted to estrogen by the liver if high enough levels occur. Estrogen can also cause breast development. Some users add other drugs to combat the side effects of anabolic steroids.

Steroid misuse quickly followed availability. During World War II, German soldiers were treated with testosterone to increase their combativeness; Russian powerlifters took so much testosterone preparing for the 1950s Olympics that urination was impossible due to drug-induced prostate gland overgrowth. Steroid abuse and its consequences were first recognized in the "anti-doping" laws adopted by the Olympic Committee in the 1960s. Anabolic steroids recently became designated as controlled substances; that is, substances with abuse potential whose access, manufacture, and distribution are regulated by law. Additional (uncontrolled) drugs that may give similar anabolic effects are already in use and may increase in use. One, gamma-hydroxybutyrate, or GHB, is a naturally-occurring brain chemical that may act as a neurotransmitter. GHB is of interest to steroid users because it reportedly releases the anabolic growth hormone. GHB is related to the inhibitory neurotransmitter, GABA, and is found together with GABA in the brain. GHB stimulates the reward circuit and has been used alone and also in a mixture with amphetamines (MAX cocktail). Serious side-effects, including seizures, coma, and death, have earned GHB the alternate nickname of "great bodily harm"; these side-effects also caused its removal from health food stores and easy, legal access.

While the mechanisms for steroid effects are known, it is still debatable whether they can significantly improve performance. This is mostly due to lack of adequately designed studies. The frequency and intensity of side-effects are unclear for similar reasons. There is also ongoing debate concerning whether tolerance and dependence occur for steroids as they do for other abused drugs. Self-administration for non-medical reasons produces a sense of well-being, if not overt euphoria. Withdrawal symptoms, including depression, restlessness, and drug-craving, have been reported. Naloxone, a narcotic-receptor antagonist (a drug that reverses the effects of narcotics), caused withdrawal-like symptoms in users of steroids only. This suggests the involvement of naturally-occurring morphine-like chemicals, and the reward circuit, in steroid dependence.

The medical uses of steroids are limited. In addition to replacement therapy, steroids may be used to treat certain cancers and anemias that do not respond to usual treatments. They are also used to stimulate appetite in the elderly and debilitated. The steroids and doses used for most medical purposes produce limited side-effects, although there are exceptions. One exception concerns use of sex steroids as anti-tumor drugs. In this case, the strategy is to remove and oppose effects of the hormone that usually affects the particular tumor tissue. For example, with certain breast cancers, the ovaries are removed and a testosterone-like steroid is given; masculinizing side-effects such as beard growth and pattern baldness usually occur at doses needed to inhibit tumor growth.

Doses of cortisol-like steroids required to suppress inflammation and/or immune responses can be very high and extend over long times. The catabolic and other effects can be very significant in such cases.

Anabolic steroids are commonly self-administered in doses high enough to produce significant side-effects, although they may be taken in cycles rather than continuously to attempt to keep these to a minimum. Doses in a cycle are increased and decreased gradually, a process known as pyramiding. Several different anabolics, oral and inject-able, may be used simultaneously, a process known as stacking, to obtain a theoretical range of different effects and in the hopes of minimizing side-effects.

How Steroids Produce Effects

1 Steroid receptors, unlike most other receptors, are located inside cells, in the fluid or cytoplasm. Steroids travel in blood bound to protein. The protein-bound steroid acts as a reservoir. This binding increases the amount of lipid-soluble steroid that can be present in blood. Because steroids are very soluble in lipid (fat), they readily enter cells from blood. Inside cells, steroids combine with their receptors. The steroids and receptors then enter the cell nucleus and interact with genetic material (DNA) to change the amount of a particular protein(s) that is made. For anabolic steroids acting on muscle cells, this might mean an increase in actin and myosin, proteins required for muscle function.

Steroid

Intracellular cytoplasmic receptor

Nucleus

DNA

Nucleolus

Nuclear pores

Ribosome

New protein

Motor neuron

● = **Acetylcholine vesicle**

Ca

Muscle fiber

2 A *muscle* is a functional group of muscle cells that usually has mostly one of two possible types of fibers, glycolytic or oxidative. The fiber types differ in oxygen requirements, glucose use, the type of exercise in which the fibers are used, and also their response to exercise training.

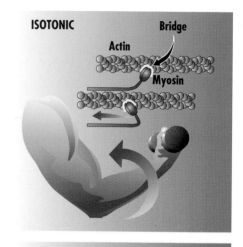

ISOTONIC

Bridge

Actin

Myosin

ISOMETRIC

6 An actual shortening of the muscle, or contraction, occurs with increased tone if the load against which the muscle is contracting is not too great; this is an isotonic contraction. As a new bridge forms between the actin and myosin, myosin pulls actin a short distance before the bridge breaks. When this happens, myosin attaches to a new site and the cycle repeats.

7 If the load is very large, the muscle may not shorten, even though additional bridges are formed and tone increases; this is an isometric contraction. For any contraction, calcium levels and muscle tone decrease as interaction between acetylcholine and its receptors stops. Bridge formation and breakage, and also return of calcium to storage, require energy that is derived from metabolism.

5 Muscle cells, like neurons, are excitable. Signals from the brain are relayed to the spinal cord where the cell bodies of motor neurons occur. Stimulation of motor neurons causes release of the neurotransmitter acetylcholine from their axon terminals. Acetylcholine, through receptors, causes an action potential in the muscle cells and increases calcium. Calcium allows the proteins actin and myosin to form temporary bridges, resulting in increased muscle tone. The maximum tone that can occur is influenced not only by the signal received by means of the action potential, but also by the amounts of actin and myosin that are present. Actin and myosin can increase in glycolytic fibers with exercise training, and may increase more with anabolic steroids if a training plateau has occurred. This is not true of oxidative fibers.

8 Testosterone regulates its own levels through a feedback relationship with the brain. Gonadotropin releasing hormone (GnRH) from the hypothalamus acts on the pituitary gland, which releases two gonadotropins, follicle stimulating hormone (FSH) and luteining hormone (LH). LH stimulates testicular Leydig cells to make testosterone, which increases in blood and locally in the testes. FSH, with testosterone, stimulates testicular support cells. FSH and testosterone are also involved in the formation and maturation of sperm. Blood testosterone is monitored, and ultimately controlled, at the hypothalamus and pituitary: *increases* in testosterone *decrease* GnRH, LH, and FSH release; a *decrease* in testosterone will *increase* GnRH, LH, and FSH. Anabolic steroids also participate in the feedback loop to the brain, decreasing GnRH, LH, and testosterone.

3 Glycolytic fibers are large in diameter. They metabolize glucose and generate (limited) energy in the form of the compound ATP. These fibers do not require much oxygen. Glycolytic muscles have fast response times, fatigue very quickly, and are used in weight- or power-lifting. Some muscles respond to exercise by increasing in size; other muscles undergo essentially invisible cellular and biochemical changes. Glycolytic muscles, also called white muscles because of their pale coloration, increase in size with training, sometimes dramatically. The increase in muscle size occurs by addition of various proteins within existing individual fibers, a mechanism potentially responsive to anabolic steroids. This potential, and the fact that glycolytic muscles are prominent "image muscles," explains the significantly greater use of anabolics by weight- and power-lifters and other athletes whose sports involve repeated fast power actions.

4 Oxidative fibers can generate large amounts of energy (ATP) from glucose. Oxidative fibers have smaller diameters than glycolytic fibers. They also contain myoglobin, an oxygen-attracting protein that is similar to hemoglobin in red blood cells, and numerous mitochondria, which are the cellular organelles in which energy from glucose is converted to ATP. This conversion relies on a sequence that uses oxygen at the last step. Oxidative muscles, also called red muscles because of their blood-like color, have slow-to-intermediate response times and fatigue slowly; they are used in endurance activities such as maintaining posture, aerobic exercise, and long distance running. Oxidative muscles do not increase much in size with training, although performance does increase due to the growth of additional blood vessels and increased blood flow. These factors improve oxygen and glucose delivery to cells that also have increased mitochondria to use them as a result of training. These changes are not very responsive to anabolic steroids, paralleling low use among athletes whose sports involve mainly repetitive endurance actions.

9 Steroids may produce adverse effects in other body systems. Increased oil secretion may contribute to seborrhea and acne, which can be severe and scarring. Inhibition of cell division can structurally weaken skin, promoting striae, or stretch marks. Body hair growth is stimulated, which can become a cosmetic problem.

The risk of cardiovascular disease may increase from a decrease in the HDL (good)/LDL (bad) cholesterol ratio. Hypertrophy of the heart (left ventricle) can occur, as a direct effect and secondary to fluid accumulation and/or increased blood pressure. Heart attacks (and also strokes), even in very young users, have been reported. The mechanism(s) are not fully documented, but possibilities include increased blood platelet reactivity and blood vessel spasm.

Steroids are metabolized in the liver. Changes in liver function, causing jaundice (yellowing of the skin), can occur, especially for high doses and oral administration. There may be an increased incidence of liver tumors, including malignant tumors, but documentation is incomplete and mechanisms are unclear. Liver metabolism of other drugs can be affected also.

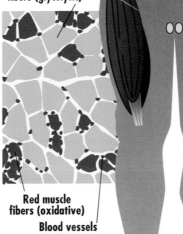
Hypothalamus releases GnRH / Pituatary gland releases FSH, LH / Hypertrophy of left heart ventricle / Liver tumors; jaundice / Testosterone / White muscle fibers (glycolytic) / Red muscle fibers (oxidative) / Blood vessels

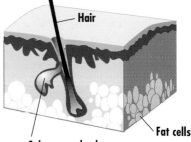
Hair / Sebaceous gland / Fat cells

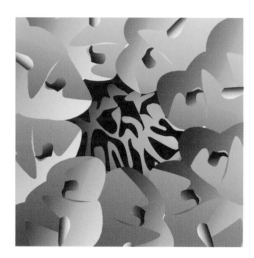

CHAPTER

Uncommon and Legal Drugs: How They Work

NUMEROUS SYNTHETIC COMPOUNDS and also naturally occurring chemicals in plants and fungi can cause hallucinations. Some of the better known examples have been discussed in previous chapters of this section, including marijuana, mushrooms, LSD, PCP, and steroids. This chapter covers several additional examples, but there are many more.

The belladona alkaloids are the compounds atropine and scopolamine. Alkaloids are nitrogen-containing substances that are present in plants. Atropine and scopolamine, and additional active derivatives, are present in many plants, including *Atropa belladonna*, *Hyoscyamus niger* (henbane), *Mandragora officinalis* (mandragora or mandrake), and *Datura stramonium* (jimson or Jamestown weed). The word *belladonna* means pretty lady. It described the dilated-pupil look that resulted from use of the plant that was considered attractive in women in the past. Poisons based on these compounds were popular in the Roman Empire, although they do not cause death easily. These and related alkaloids were the active ingredients in witches' ointments. Australian aborigines use corkwood, which contains significant amounts of atropine, scopolamine, and related compounds, to stun and capture fish. These compounds have medical uses as well.

Atropine and scopolamine produce effects by blocking the subset of receptors for the neuro-transmitter acetylcholine that can be stimulated with the mushroom toxin muscarine. These effects take place in the central nervous system (CNS) and in the peripheral nervous system (PNS), and they last for up to 48 hours. CNS effects include hallucinations, specifically involving flying, and also amnesia. Effects in the PNS include dry mouth, high body temperature without perspiration, dilation of skin blood vessels, and increased heart rate. Unlike other hallucinogens, the belladona alkaloids apparently produce at least one recurrent and predictable hallucination, that of flying. Flight hallucinations were also prominent features of Native American rituals in which *Datura stramonium* was used. *Datura* species contain significant amounts of belladonna alkaloids.

Mescaline is the hallucinogenic compound contained in the small, globular southwestern mescal cactus, *Lophophora williamsii*. The name *mescaline* indicates its identification with the Mescalero Apaches, whose religious rites involved its use. Sections of the cactus's top are dried to produce mescal buttons, also known as peyotl or peyote. The dried buttons are consumed to produce drug effects, which can last up to 12 hours after a single dose. Mescaline has a chemical structure (identified in 1918) most closely related to the neurotransmitter norepinephrine and to the amphetamines, particularly hallucinogenic designer amphetamines such as MDA. However, mescaline effects most closely resemble those of LSD. These effects include vivid visual hallucinations, altered color and space perception, and signs of stimulation of the sympathetic nervous system (increased heart rate, for example). Mescaline is less potent than psilocin and much less potent than LSD. There is cross tolerance between LSD and mescaline, and also psilocin, supporting the similarity of mechanism as well as effect among them.

Nutmeg and mace are examples of ordinary substances that can produce hallucinations. For example, the fruit (nut) of the tree *Myristica fragrans* provides two familiar spices: the coating on the shell provides mace and the nutmeat provides nutmeg. Most people are familiar with the uses and flavors of these spices. Less familiar are the hallucinogenic effects of both spices, due to two weakly active compounds, myristicin and elemicin. The chemical structures of both are, like mescaline, similar to norepinephrine or the designer amphetamines, while the effects are more like LSD. Often one of these spices is used when preferred substances are unavailable. In order to obtain hallucinogenic effects, at least two whole nutmegs must be ground and extracted (as a tea, for example). Once drunk, there may be a lengthy delay before effects start. Gastrointestinal side effects are apparently unpleasant enough to deter frequent use.

Morning glories can be used to produce *ololiuqui*, a mildly hallucinogenic South American beverage. Seeds from *Ipomoea* species morning glories provide the active ingredient. Ololiuqui was analyzed prior to the preparation of LSD and was found to contain lysergic acid amide (LSA), a simpler and weaker derivative of lysergic acid than LSD. Seeds of many common morning glories contain this compound, which can be extracted from them after cracking or grinding. LSA also occurs in association with other plants, for example, sleepy weed (*Stipa robusta*), an invader of western grazing areas that can sedate horses for up to a week. The LSA is actually produced by a fungus (*Acremonium*) that lives on the grass, reminiscent of the lysergic acid compounds that can occur on rye grain during an infection by the ergot fungus (*Claviceps purpurea*).

Toads are often ingredients in "magic" potions, as are toadstools (poisonous mushrooms). For a time, the hallucinogenic mushroom *Amanita muscaria* was thought to produce its effects through the compound bufotenin, which is also found in the skin of certain toads. The chemical structure of bufotenin is similar to that of the neurotransmitter serotonin, and to LSD. Bufotenin does produce hallucinations, but it is not involved in the effects of *Amanita muscaria*, which contains negligible amounts, if any, of the compound. Tales of hallucinations resulting from toad abuse—for example, toad licking—have been labeled suspect, since the amount of bufotenin in or on toad skin is probably too low to produce any effect. Despite this, toads were recently added to the list of controlled substances; possessing or using toads can result in fines and/or imprisonment.

How Various Hallucinogens Work

Atropine occurs in high amounts in *Atropa belladonna*, a plant native to Europe that now grows wild in the United States. The berries are sweet (which poses an attractive risk to children in particular) but especially high in atropine. *Hyoscyamus niger* contains high amounts of scopolamine.

Atropa belladonna

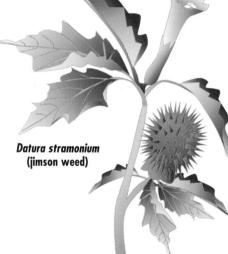

Datura stramonium (jimson weed)

Datura stramonium is native to North America. All parts of the plant contain significant amounts of atropine, scopolamine, and related compounds. *Datura* species have been used in Native American rituals. An early incident in Jamestown, Virginia resulted in its alternate name, jimson or Jamestown weed. Soldiers who were sent to Jamestown to quell a disturbance were rendered incoherent for nearly two weeks when *Datura* was inadvertently included in their food.

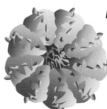

Lophophora williamsii (mescaline, peyote)

The mescal cactus has been a part of rituals for indigenous populations from Central America throughout the southwestern United States. Peyote is still used, legally, in various Indian rituals. It is a recognized sacrament of the Native American Church.

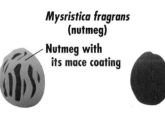

Mysristica fragrans (nutmeg)

Nutmeg with its mace coating

Nutmeg and mace both contain the hallucinogenic chemicals myristicin and elemicin. The chemical structures of both are, like mescaline, similar to norepinephrine or the designer amphetamines, while the effects are more like LSD. Use of either spice often occurs when preferred substances are unavailable.

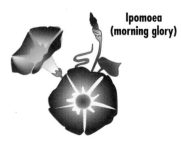

Ipomoea (morning glory)

Morning glories are widely distributed. The names of some, for example Heavenly Blue, may indicate their hallucinogenic potential. The seeds contain most of the hallucinogenic chemicals.

The compounds atropine and scopolamine, and numerous related compounds, can block the effect of the neurotransmitter acetylcholine on some of its receptors. Specifically, the subset of receptors stimulated by muscarine are affected. Muscarine is chemically similar to acetylcholine and is found in some hallucinogenic mushrooms. Acetylcholine functions in many brain areas, particularly those involved with memory and movement. Acetylcholine is also present in the peripheral nervous system. Its actions on glands and organs are mediated through muscarinic receptors; its actions in other sites are mediated by nicotinic receptors, that is, receptors that can be stimulated by acetylcholine or nicotine. Blockade of central acetylcholine receptors results in sedation, confusion, hallucinations, and amnesia.

There is no re-uptake for acetylcholine; it is degraded by a postsynaptic enzyme, which halts its action.

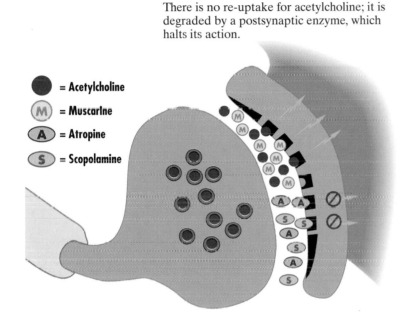

- ● = Acetylcholine
- Ⓜ = Muscarine
- Ⓐ = Atropine
- Ⓢ = Scopolamine

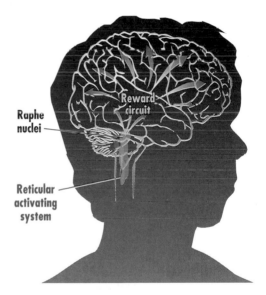

Raphe nuclei

Reward circuit

Reticular activating system

The effects of many hallucinogenic plants resemble the effects of LSD. The individual compounds responsible are often chemically very similar to the neurotransmitter serotonin. Some exceptions include the active compounds in other hallucinogenic plants that are more closely related to the neurotransmitter norepinephrine and some amphetamines, specifically the designer amphetamines derived from methamphetamine—for example, MDA and MDMA. Despite this difference in structure, the effects of these compounds closely resemble those of LSD, which affects the raphe nuclei of the reticular activating system (RAS). The various hallucinogenic compounds differ mainly in potency, not in effect and not in mechanism of producing effect.

Sources of Information and Assistance

Included here are several comprehensive sources that can provide not only information about individual drugs, but also phone numbers, addresses, and more for state and local agencies that you can contact for additional information or services. The following directories are usually available in the government documents section of public libraries. They also may be obtained at nominal costs from the Government Printing Office (GPO), or single copies may be available without cost from the National Clearinghouse for Alcohol and Drug Abuse Information (NCADI: 1-800-729-6686).

In addition to these directories, listings of some hotlines and agencies for specific drugs or specific groups are available; where appropriate, document numbers are also provided. Tollfree numbers are included for most of them. In general, local telephone directories have fairly comprehensive listings, so this source should not be overlooked or dismissed. Local newspapers also publish schedules for meetings of local affiliates of national agencies; these announcements will typically provide names and telephone contacts. Local health providers, religious groups, and government offices are other sources of information.

Comprehensive Directories

Citizen's Alcohol and Other Drug Prevention Directory: Resources for Getting Involved. Office for Substance Abuse Prevention (OSAP), 5600 Fishers Lane, Rockville, MD 20857. DHHS (Department of Health and Human Services) Publication # (ADM) 90-1657 1990. Includes individual listings by federal and national agencies, as well as by states and territories. It also lists clearinghouses and resource centers.

National Directory of Drug Abuse and Alcoholism Treatment and Prevention Programs. Office of Applied Studies, 5600 Fishers Lane, Rockwall II, Suite 615, Rockville, MD 20857. DHHS Publication # (SMA) 93-2050 1993. There are 11,632 programs listed, with a comprehensive key for services offered.

Hotlines, Helplines, Specific Drug Lines

Alcoholics Anonymous (AA). Information and support are provided through local chapters nationwide. Consult your telephone directory.

Al-Anon/Alateen. 1-800-443-4525; 1-800-356-9996 for brochure. Provides information on alcoholism and alcohol abuse and referrals to local Al-Anon and Alateen support groups for friends and families of alcoholics.

American Council for Drug Education. 1-800-488-3784. Provides brochures.

American Council on Alcoholism Helpline. 1-800-527-5344. Services include referrals to alcohol treatment programs nationwide and access to written materials.

Center for Substance Abuse Treatment. 1-800-622-4357. Provides local referrals.

Children of Alcoholics Foundation, Inc. 1-800-359-2623. Provides reports, brochures, referrals, and preview videos.

Cocaine Anonymous (CA). 1-800-347-8998. Provides nationwide referrals, 24 hours a day.

Drug Abuse Information and Treatment Hotline (NIDA). 1-800-662-4357 or (Spanish) 1-800-662-9832. This federally funded service provides referrals to drug and alcohol programs, including referrals to programs for those who cannot pay.

Drug-Free Workplace Helpline (CSAP/NIDA). 1-800-843-4971. Provides individualized technical assistance to businesses, industry, and unions on drug-free workplace programs, including employee education, supervisor training, and signs and symptoms of drug abuse.

International Institute for Inhalant Abuse. 1-800-832-5090. This is a clearinghouse for information, providing print materials, referrals, and education.

Kidsrights. 1-800-892-5437. Provides print materials and referrals.

Narcotics Anonymous (NA). 1-818-780-3951. Information and support are provided through local chapters nationwide. Consult your telephone directory.

Nar-Anon. 1-310-547-5800. Similar to Al-Anon, but for friends and families of drug users. Provides referrals.

National Association of State Alcohol and Drug Abuse Directors (NASADAD). 1-202-783-6868. Coordinates federal and state agencies. Also a resource on state drug programs, providing contacts in each state.

National Cancer Institute. 1-800-422-6237. Provides additional tobacco and health information.

National Clearinghouse for Alcohol and Drug Abuse Information (NCADI). 1-800-729-6686. Provides latest research results, popular press and scientific journal articles, videos, prevention curricula, print materials, program descriptions, state-level contacts, and RADAR (Regional Alcohol and Drug Awareness) center contacts and phone numbers.

National Council on Alcoholism and Drug Dependency (NCADD) Helpline. 1-800-622-2255. Provides information on alcohol abuse, referrals to treatment and counseling centers across the country; 7 days a week, 24 hours a day.

National Hotline. 1-800-262-2463. Information and referrals to drug rehabilitation and counseling services within its area; also provides cocaine and crack information by mail.

National Institute for Occupational Safety and Health (NIOSH), Publications Office. 1-800-356-4674. Provides additional inhalant information.

Substance Abuse Information Database (SAID). 1-800-808-0965. Free, online database available by modem or free computer program for use on your own PC, both updated regularly; Department of Labor service for employers seeking information on substance abuse in the workplace.

USEPA Indoor Air Quality Information Clearinghouse. 1-800-438-4318. Information on second-hand tobacco smoke.

Additional Information

Drugs and Pregnancy   March of Dimes Birth Defects Foundation, 1-914-428-7100.

Drug Testing   For a current listing of labs certified by HHS to perform urine testing, contact Dr. Donna Bush, Chief, Drug Testing Section/Division of Workplace Programs SAMHSA, 1-301-443-6014. This data is also published in *The Federal Register* (updated monthly).

Drugs and Driving   National Center for Statistics and Analysis, 1-202-366-4198. Provides information on alcohol and traffic fatalities.

Address for GPO
Superintendent of Documents
Government Printing Office
Washington, DC 20402
(Include document number)